Understanding Doctors' Performance

Edited by

Jim Cox
Lead Assessor and Trainer, General Medical Council performance procedures
Former Associate Director (Assessment Development),
National Clinical Assessment Authority
Medical Director, Cumbria Ambulance Service NHS Trust

Jennifer King
Chartered Psychologist
Managing Director, Edgecumbe Consulting Group

Allen Hutchinson
Head of Section of Public Health
ScHARR, University of Sheffield

and

Pauline McAvoy
Associate Director (Assessment Development),
National Clinical Assessment Service of the National Patient Safety Agency

Radcliffe Publishing
Oxford ● Seattle

Radcliffe Publishing Ltd
18 Marcham Road
Abingdon
Oxon OX14 1AA
United Kingdom

www.radcliffe-oxford.com
Electronic catalogue and worldwide online ordering facility.

British Library Cataloguing in Publication Data

A catalogue record for this book is available from the British Library.

ISBN 1 85775 766 1

Typeset by Advance Typesetting Ltd, Oxford
Printed and bound by TJ International Ltd, Padstow, Cornwall

Contents

About the editors

Dr Jim Cox
Lead Assessor and Trainer, General Medical Council performance procedures
Former Associate Director (Assessment Development),
National Clinical Assessment Authority
Medical Director, Cumbria Ambulance Service NHS Trust

Dr Jennifer King
Chartered Psychologist
Managing Director, Edgecumbe Consulting Group

Professor Allen Hutchinson
Head of Section of Public Health
ScHARR, University of Sheffield

Professor Pauline McAvoy
Associate Director (Assessment Development),
National Clinical Assessment Service of the National Patient Safety Agency

List of contributors

Dr Carol Borrill
Senior Lecturer
University of Nottingham

Professor Jenny Firth-Cozens
Consultant
Clinical and Occupational Psychology

Dr Susanna Galea
Clinical Lecturer and Specialist Registrar in Addictive Behaviour
St George's University of London

Professor Hamid Ghodse
Professor of Psychiatry and International Drug Policy
Director, International Centre for Drug Policy
St George's University of London

Dr Kirstie Gibson
Specialist Registrar in Occupational Health
Guy's and St Thomas's NHS Trust

Dr John Harrison
Clinical Director of Occupational Health
Hammersmith Hospitals NHS Trust

Dr Luke Kartsounis
Consultant Clinical Neuropsychologist
Oldchurch Hospital

Professor Michael Kopelman
Consultant Neuropsychiatrist
St Thomas's Hospital

Professor Elisabeth Paice
Dean Director, London Deanery

Dr Lawrence Smith
School of Psychology
University of Leeds

Dr Marion Spendlove
Research Fellow, Aston Business School

Dr John Sterland
Specialist Registrar in Occupational Medicine
King's College Hospital

Professor Michael West
Professor of Organisational Psychology
Aston Business School

Acknowledgements

This book arises from the work of a group convened and sponsored by the National Clinical Assessment Authority (NCAA), now the National Clinical Assessment Service of the National Patient Safety Agency. The NCAA published a synopsis report *Understanding Performance Difficulties in Doctors* in November 2004.

The editors particularly thank Dr Rosemary Field, Deputy Director of the National Clinical Assessment Service, for her support, encouragement and advice. They are also extremely grateful to Kevin Hunt and Sheila Mariswamy, who managed the project.

Introduction

Like other health professionals, most doctors work hard, strive to achieve high standards and provide excellent services for their patients. But there are more than 100 000 practising doctors in the UK and it is inevitable that some of them fail to meet reasonable standards.

Doctors' professional performance has become the focus of unprecedented public scrutiny. Most people had assumed that their doctors were competent, but several highly publicised cases in the United Kingdom showed how that trust could sometimes be misplaced. Failings of paediatric cardiac surgeons in Bristol led the *British Medical Journal* to conclude in an editorial: 'All changed, changed utterly' (Smith, 1998).

The medical profession had begun to address the problems of poor performance of doctors before these events made headline news, but public exposure of poor performance made it more urgent to find solutions.

By 1995 the General Medical Council (GMC), the body responsible for regulation of the medical profession, had obtained the necessary legislative framework to introduce 'Performance Procedures' which allow them to investigate and, if necessary, restrict the practice of doctors who may be putting their patients or the public at risk. The GMC developed methods to assess both competence (what the doctor *can* do) and performance (what the doctor *does* do) (Southgate *et al.*, 2001) which have been sufficiently robust to withstand legal challenge. GMC performance assessments, quite properly since they are intended to protect the public, concentrate on *description* of the doctor's clinical performance with reference to current standards. They are not designed to explain *why* the doctor's performance is substandard. Furthermore, the GMC has tended to concentrate its work at the extreme end of the spectrum of poor performance, with procedures which are more disciplinary than developmental.

In 2001 the National Clinical Assessment Authority (now part of the National Patient Safety Agency) was created as a special Health Authority of the National Health Service (NHS) to advise the NHS about the management of poor performance. Its stated aim was 'promoting confidence in doctors and dentists' (NCAA, 2004a). Like the GMC, it undertakes assessments of performance but, unlike the GMC, its assessments are formative, intended to clarify concerns and to make recommendations to the doctor and the NHS body to whom the doctor is responsible. As well as assessing clinical performance, an assessment includes, as a matter of routine, psychometric testing, an interview with a behavioural psychologist and assessment by an occupational health physician. The thrust of these assessments – and the impetus for this book – is to try to *explain* the doctor's practice as well as to describe it. Understanding more about the possible causes of a doctor's practice helps to inform the most appropriate recommendations or remediation.

Regulators and other interested parties in other countries, particularly Australia, New Zealand, Canada and the USA are also working on the same problems. In general, there are three levels of assessment: screening whole populations of doctors (level 1), the targeting of 'at risk' groups (level 2) and assessing individual practitioners who may be performing poorly (level 3) (Finucane PM *et al.*, 2003). Canadian provinces, for example, have a number of well-developed level 1 (screening) and level 2 (targeted assessment) programmes. Although level 3 performance assessments carried out in the UK are widely acknowledged as being the most highly developed in the world, so far we have no well-developed system for level 1 or level 2 assessments in the UK. They are likely to be introduced in the near future as part of the proposals for regular revalidation of doctors. The assessment of the factors described in this book would usually be part of a level 3 assessment but, of course, the causes of poor performance are the same however they are assessed.

One of the most significant changes to affect the medical profession in recent years is the recognition that being a good doctor is about more than just technical and clinical competence, skills or knowledge. The dissemination of the GMC document on the principles of Good Medical Practice (General Medical Council, 1998) has highlighted and embedded the importance of non-clinical attributes including team working, leadership, and communication. There is increasing evidence that complaints about doctors revolve largely around their behaviour (Sanger, 1998).

So what are the factors that cause a doctor who *can* practise safely not to do so? Why do some doctors successfully address their difficulties while others fail to do so? What is the impact of such factors as physical and psychological health, cognitive deterioration, personality, attitudes, values, beliefs, workload, sleep loss, shift patterns, organisational culture, teamwork, leadership and life events and so on?

Early experience of including behavioural assessment as part of performance assessment has provided some insights, as has the work of regulatory bodies in other countries such as Canada, Australia and New Zealand. For example, Canadian experience indicates that cognitive impairment may affect up to a third of poorly performing physicians assessed in Ontario (Ferguson B, personal communication). Similarly, although numbers are too small to generalise with confidence, a review of the first 50 assessments carried out by the National Clinical Assessment Authority revealed that two doctors (4%) were affected by cognitive impairment.

How widespread is poor performance amongst doctors? The international literature has shown consistently for more than a decade that in the hospital workforce there are around 6% of doctors with serious performance problems (Donaldson, 1994). Of those whose performance has been assessed by one of the national bodies, only a small minority are simply incompetent.

The themes of this book were first presented as a report for the NHS (NCAA, 2004b). We believe that this is the first time anyone has attempted to bring together existing knowledge about the factors influencing a doctor's performance. Our aim is to provide practical, evidence-based guidance to assist individuals, employers and regulatory, educational and professional agencies that are faced with the challenge of managing concerns about the performance of doctors. Although the primary focus is on doctors, many of the issues are equally applicable to other health professionals, including dentists.

Our initial literature search revealed a complex array of issues that can impact on a doctor's performance. Some clear themes emerged and these provide the basis for our chapter headings. Some themes, whilst crucially important, proved difficult to cover satisfactorily in a single chapter – in particular, issues concerning ethnicity, equality and diversity. These cut across many different topic areas. Rather than risk oversimplifying issues of such sensitivity and significance we chose to address them, as appropriate, as part of a number of chapters. There is a substantial and broad-ranging international literature on the impact of ethnicity and diversity on human performance and, to a lesser extent, on the performance of healthcare staff. Much of the literature concludes that inequalities that impact on minority groups exist around the world, in the whole field of human endeavour.

Similarly, there is an extensive literature on safety and quality issues in healthcare which lies beyond the scope of this book but which we recognise is central to the issues relating to poor performance in doctors. Finally, although some high-profile cases concern criminal or unethical activities, we have not addressed them in this book. Procedures for dealing with them do not normally include performance assessment.

Chapters in the book were commissioned from experts who were asked to review and analyse the relevant literature and address specific questions to develop our understanding of the significance, assessment and possible remediation of factors that affect performance. Each contribution was further refined by discussion and editing by the working group.

We aimed to answer some important practical questions about each of the factors identified:

- What are the factors that influence a doctor's performance?
- Why do the factors arise?
- To what extent does each factor affect performance?
- What are the most effective methods for assessing each factor and its impact on the performance of a doctor?
- To what extent does each factor affect the remediability of poor performance?
- For which factors has intervention been effective?
- How sustainable are changes which result from interventions likely to be?
- What are the questions for further research?

We are aware of many of the limitations of this exercise (and, no doubt, ignorant of others). Nevertheless, we hope that this work will be a useful contribution to the world literature on performance assessment and be of interest to regulators and professions other than medicine in the UK and abroad. In the longer term we hope that the insights gained from this work will help us to promote and restore confidence in our doctors.

References

Donaldson LJ (1994) Doctors with problems in an NHS workforce. *BMJ.* **308**: 1277–82.

Ferguson B. Personal communication.

Finucane PM, Bourgeois-Law GA, Ineson SL and Kaigas TM (2003) A comparison of performance assessment programs for medical practitioners in Canada, Australia, New Zealand, and the United Kingdom. *Acad Med.* **78**(8): 837–43.

General Medical Council (1998) *Good Medical Practice*. General Medical Council, London.

NCAA (2004a) *NCAA Handbook*. NCAA, London.

NCAA (2004b) Understanding performance difficulties in doctors. NCAA, London.

Sanger J (1998) Putting the person in the appraisal. *Clin in Mgmt.* **9**: 195.

Smith R (1998) All changed, changed utterly. *BMJ.* **316**: 1917–18.

Southgate L, Cox J, David T *et al.* (2001) The assessment of poorly performing doctors: the development of the assessment programmes for the General Medical Council's performance procedures. *Med Educ.* **35**(Suppl 1): 2–8.

Chapter 1

The impact of health on performance

John Harrison and John Sterland

Introduction

There are few published studies on doctors' physical illnesses. Although doctors are more vulnerable than others to psychological and psychiatric problems, it does not appear that they are troubled by physical illness any more than are other people. That is not to say that physical illnesses do not occur in doctors. A *State of the Art Review* (Emmett, 1987) identifies infectious diseases, chemical agents, musculo-skeletal problems and stress as important occupational health issues for healthcare workers in general. Most problems are exposure-specific. The Royal College of Physicians, in association with the Faculty of Occupational Medicine, published a report concerned with health risks to the healthcare professional (Litchfield, 1995). Chapters on blood-borne viruses, tuberculosis and allergic respiratory disease were concerned with healthcare workers in general; chapters on mental ill health, burnout and alcohol problems were concerned with doctors in particular.

The context of this review is the relationship between diseases in doctors and their performance at work. The management of a surgeon infected with hepatitis B virus is relatively straightforward in that there are objective tests for hepatitis B surface antigen and there is clear guidance about fitness to perform exposure-prone procedures (Department of Health, 2000). On the other hand, the management of a doctor whose behaviour is at variance from a perceived norm, or whose decision-making processes are unusual, is more difficult because of the professional inde-pendence of specialists and principals in general practice. This may be compounded by doctors' attitudes to their own health and an unwillingness to behave like other patients. Unfortunately, such important topics have only recently become research areas.

Any significant medical problem that affects judgement and performance can compromise a doctor's ability to provide good medical care. The American Medical Association defines an impaired physician as 'one unable to fulfil professional or personal responsibilities because of psychiatric illness, alcoholism or drug depend-ency' (Boisaubin & Levine, 2001). It is estimated that approximately 15% of physicians will be impaired at some point in their careers. In a recent review of evidence of ill health in the medical profession in the United Kingdom only 1% of doctors who were referred to the General Medical Council's (GMC) health committee had a problem with physical health (Stanton & Caan, 2003). General Medical Council records show that 199 out of 201 doctors under supervision at the end of 2001 had problems with alcohol, drugs or mental ill health.

In contrast to GMC referrals, reasons for ill health retirement include a greater proportion of doctors with physical, rather than psychological, illness. The com-monest reasons for doctors taking early retirement from the National Health Service are psychiatric (33%), musculo-skeletal (27%) and cardiovascular (17%) illnesses (Pattani, Constantinovici & Williams, 2001). Perhaps it is easier for doctors with physical problems to admit that there is a problem, particularly if the job is of a manual nature (such as in the interventionist specialties) so that the symptoms are obviously disabling. It might also be expected that doctors will have better insight into the implications of these illnesses with respect to their fitness for work. This may not be the case when the problem is substance abuse or depression. Pension scheme rules are also a factor, in that physical illnesses might be more likely to be assessed as causing permanent ill health.

Because of the paucity of published data on physical illnesses in doctors, the first part of this chapter considers the potential effects of physical illnesses on judgement and performance and how they might be assessed. Doctors' attitudes and behaviour in respect of their own health and wellbeing are also explored. Where possible, we discuss the potential for occupational health interventions and improvement in performance. This is consistent with an occupational health approach to the assessment of fitness for work. This comprises a clinical evaluation of a worker, taking into account the activities of the job and associated risks to health and safety, either to the individual worker, other workers or to third parties. In the case of doctors, the third parties include patients. Thus, impaired performance of a surgeon may be affected by the onset of a Parkinsonian tremor affecting a hand, whereas a similar tremor in a public health physician may have less relevance in terms of fitness for work.

Some physical illnesses can lead to cognitive impairment or co-existent psychiatric illness. These are also discussed, but cognitive impairment is covered in more detail in Chapter 4.

Chronic illness and disability

A comprehensive review of the health of healthcare workers, including ill health amongst doctors, was carried out on behalf of a partnership of organisations convened by the Nuffield Trust (Williams, Michie & Pattani, 1998). The major findings were of ill health related to psychological disturbances and unhealthy lifestyles, including excessive alcohol consumption. The review referred to a survey of junior doctors indicating that they tended to report frequent minor illnesses, but that they rarely took time off work. Self-prescription was common. Back pain was a feature in nurses, but not in doctors. Cardiovascular disease was not reported by either doctors or nurses.

A recent attempt to quantify how many doctors are sick (Stanton & Caan, 2003) combined a literature search with an enquiry of organisations including the Department of Health and the GMC, and care organisations such as the National Counselling Service for Sick Doctors. Not surprisingly, the results reinforced the impression that psychiatric illness is the main affliction of doctors. It was noted that calls for help about drugs and alcohol had reduced in recent years. This was felt to be an indication of a reluctance on the part of doctors to seek help rather than a decrease in the incidence of addicted doctors.

Shift-working for more than 6 years has been suggested as a risk factor for coronary heart disease in nurses, albeit probably as a result of the combined effects of smoking, increased body mass index, low levels of activity, hypertension and diabetes (Stanton & Caan, 2003).

Doctors have low mortality rates (Carpenter, Swerdlow & Fear, 1997). NHS hospital consultants had less than half the mortality rate expected for the period 1962 to 1979. Low mortality was found for cardiovascular disease, lung cancer and other smoking-related diseases and for diabetes. Studies show excess mortality for doctors in overdose of prescribed drugs and suicide in female doctors. A significant excess mortality in anaesthetists from cirrhosis of the liver was felt to merit further study. Other mortality studies have looked at deaths from smoking (Doll *et al.*, 1994a) and alcohol (Doll *et al.*, 1994b). Excess mortality from smoking-related diseases was found between 1971 and 1991, compared to that between 1951 and 1971. However, those doctors that stopped smoking before middle age had virtually no increased risk of mortality from smoking-related diseases. The now well-known 'U'-shaped curve relationship concerning all-cause mortality and the average amount of alcohol reportedly drunk showing that a little alcohol is more beneficial than none, but that excess alcohol increases risk, was first discovered in a study of male British doctors.

There is some information on physical illnesses occurring in junior doctors. A dedicated occupational health service in the north-east of England has taken referrals of junior doctors with health problems since 1996 (Harrison & Redfern, 2001). Unpublished data reveal that doctors had a wide range of physical illnesses, including diabetes, epilepsy, multiple sclerosis, asthma, low back pain, osteoarthritis, ulcerative colitis, viral meningitis, neuropraxia, Hodgkin's disease and polycystic ovaries.

Further information about disabilities experienced by medical students and doctors comes from a survey of deans of medical schools, postgraduate deans, associate postgraduate deans and regional advisors in general practice carried out by a working party convened by the British Medical Association (BMA) (British Medical Association, 1997). A long list of physical diseases was collated. The conditions reported most frequently were paraplegia, hearing impairment, multiple sclerosis, visual impairment, hemiplegia and epilepsy. More than half of the respondents had their condition prior to, or developed the condition during, training at medical school. Disability was defined as the end result of physical, mental or sensory impairment, or long-term ill health (which can limit functional ability). Either case may result in loss or limitation of opportunities. Impairment does not imply being unable to fulfil professional responsibilities, although it may occur if suitable adjustments to the working environment are not made, or if workplace attitudes militate against effective practice.

Some important chronic diseases and their effects

Diabetes mellitus is a common chronic condition which can affect doctors like everyone else. It is referred to as an unseen disability (Hirst, 2003). It is not a contraindication to clinical practice, but doctors working night shifts, or long and stressful hours, and not eating properly and regularly must overcome problems of glycaemic control. Working with low blood sugars at some point is almost inevitable. Some people with diabetes do not have warning signs of hypoglycaemic attacks and so may compensate by allowing their blood sugars to run higher than normal.

Occasionally, symptoms associated with poor glycaemic control, such as fatigue or impaired performance during operating theatre sessions or in other safety-critical areas of practice, may require occupational health support to modify hours of work and activities undertaken. Loss of control may be a temporary phenomenon and support from colleagues is required during this period. It is helpful if a doctor's colleagues are aware of the diagnosis, although this has to be handled sensitively. The doctor concerned has to be prepared to accept help and to acknowledge that they are not always in control of their own health.

Epilepsy is another relatively common chronic illness that requires an occupational health assessment of fitness for practice. Unfortunately, there is still a stigma attached to the diagnosis of epilepsy that can discourage doctors from admitting the problem to their colleagues, let alone to patients. Although infrequent seizures may not unduly affect a doctor's ability to practise, frequent seizures can be very disruptive to the delivery of care, especially in an era of intense pressure to meet clinical targets. Once again the main concern relates to safety-critical jobs. Considerations such as lone working and driving are important particularly if, for example, doctors are on call and attend urgent clinical cases alone.

The duration and nature of the aura are important. If there is sufficient warning before the onset of a seizure, most areas of practice can be considered. The frequency and nature of seizures are also important, as are any identified triggers. As well as affecting the victim, tonic-clonic seizures can be disturbing to other health workers.

If there is sufficient warning the doctor can go to a quiet area before the onset of the seizure. It is important that others around ensure that no harm results and that they are trained to realise that there is no need to panic or to intervene unnecessarily and that, after the seizure, the doctor will feel drowsy and may wish to sleep for several hours.

Complex partial seizures may manifest themselves as absences or automatic behaviour. During their occurrence the doctor may be unresponsive to questions or instructions. This can be unsettling for patients, carers or, in paediatrics, parents.

Multiple sclerosis is relatively common, usually beginning in the early years of working life. In any deanery or NHS region it is likely that there will be several junior doctors and two or three career grade doctors, either in hospital practice or in general practice, with the condition. Its nature is variable. Relapses may occur intermittently, causing periods of temporary unfitness followed by long periods of fitness to practise. Other cases progress more steadily.

Problems with eyesight, mobility and/or co-ordination are typical occupational health issues to be addressed. Adjustments can be made to assist doctors with mobility problems including the provision of electric vehicles for moving around hospitals. Upper limb ataxia may be a more significant disability. In one case a junior doctor in paediatrics was able to continue in clinical practice despite lower limb problems, but when her left arm became affected she had to give up routine practice and adopt a teaching role. Some doctors with multiple sclerosis lack insight into how badly they are affected. In such cases it is necessary to confront them with their problems in as sympathetic a manner as possible. It is also important to see the wider picture, not just the disability. Attitudes of peers and seniors are very important.

Parkinson's disease presents later in life and is unusual in junior doctors. Typically it will present in a hospital consultant or a GP principal. The four cardinal signs of Parkinson's disease – tremor, rigidity, slowness and difficulty in starting and stopping walking – contribute to the disabilities of the illness (Marsden, 2000). The patient 'shuffles', handwriting becomes small and untidy and rapid movements of hands and feet are impaired. Drug therapy can control symptoms initially, but may cause long-term problems. Such problems mean that continuing to practise medicine after the diagnosis has been made is unlikely unless a new restricted role is available. Surgeons normally have to cease to operate once the diagnosis has been confirmed, even if their symptoms can be controlled by medication. From a clinical governance perspective, the risk to patients of an adverse outcome due to failure to control symptoms, albeit intermittently, is too great.

During excerbations, **ulcerative colitis** can cause malaise and tiredness as well as the need to leave the workplace to use the toilet. Associated conditions, such as uveitis or arthropathy can also be problematic. In addition, treatment of severe exacerbations can cause steroid-induced behavioural changes that create difficulties if the doctor has tried to continue in clinical practice. In an extreme case, apparent abnormal behaviour caused by steroid treatment led to disciplinary proceedings.

Rheumatoid arthritis or sero-negative arthritis can interfere with clinical practice, if a doctor is required to spend a lot of time standing or walking, or must maintain set postures at work, perhaps in anaesthetics, surgery or interventional radiology. Arthritis of the hands is particularly important if manipulation of instruments is a feature of the job.

Hepatic failure may result from cirrhosis, which may be a result of alcohol abuse, or infection with hepatitis B or C virus. Hepatic encephalopathy may result from liver failure. In some cases encephalopathy is sub-clinical inasmuch as routine clinical examination is normal, but psychometric assessments reveal impaired brain function. Safety-critical jobs, such as surgery, should be avoided, unless the doctor is part of a surgical team and does not have ultimate responsibility for decision making.

Chronic renal failure Although many of the disabling symptoms associated with renal failure requiring dialysis can be counteracted by erythropoietin, there remain concerns about fitness to practise for doctors in safety-critical jobs. Glomerular filtration rates of less than 20 ml/min are usually associated with symptoms such as lassitude. Although commercial pilots would be prevented from flying (Raymond Johnston, Chief Medical Officer of the CAA – personal communication), in some cases treatment by regular nightly peritoneal dialysis may control symptoms sufficiently to permit limited work, including assisting at surgery.

Deficient vision

This has been shown to be important when assessing histopathologists (Poole *et al.*, 1997). Out of 132 doctors, 13% had colour deficient vision. Fourteen were deutan (green colour deficient) and 1 was protan (red colour deficient). Doctors with colour deficiency were significantly poorer at identifying test slides than doctors with normal colour vision. In addition, the severity of colour deficiency correlated with the number of mistakes made, including missing mycobacteria, amyloid or Helicobacter pylori.

Depression caused by physical illness

Physical illnesses associated with depression include HIV infection, neurological diseases (Parkinson's disease, Huntington's disease, epilepsy and stroke), musculo-skeletal complaints, heart disease and diabetes mellitus. A past history of depression increases the probability of recurrence of depression during medical illness.

Diagnosing depression in the physically ill can be difficult because symptoms may be due to the underlying physical illness. Strategies to counter this have been described (Parker & Kalucy, 1999) including an 'inclusive' approach (taking account of all symptoms, irrespective of cause), an 'exclusive' approach (ignoring potentially confounding features such as anorexia and fatigue) and an aetiological approach (discounting symptoms that are considered solely due to the medical condition).

A measure that has been developed to be used for people who are medically ill is the Hospital Anxiety and Depression Scale. However, simple screening measures, such as merely asking 'Are you depressed?', might be as sensitive as more complicated measures (Parker & Kalucy, 1999).

When depression is present, treatment using conventional methods can make a major impact on health and wellbeing.

Illness and behaviour

Many doctors are reluctant to see other doctors about their health. In 1995 an Australian randomised sample postal survey of doctors' attitudes towards their own medical care (with a 44% response rate) showed that whilst almost one-fifth had marital or emotional problems, 3% admitted to alcohol problems and 1% to drug problems, only 42% had a GP and few had discussed their problems with them (Pullen *et al.*, 1995). A 1999 New Zealand questionnaire study on a random sample of doctors found that although many claimed to be working under substantial stress, relatively few had regular health assessments. A case was made for regular checks (Richards, 1999). A Spanish questionnaire survey of 795 doctors showed that 49% did not have a family doctor, 82% self-prescribed and 47% did not attend occupational health appointments (Bruguera *et al.*, 2001). In a more recent 2003 Australian study of 896 doctors with a 40% response rate, 90% said that self-treatment of acute conditions was acceptable and 25% would self-prescribe for a chronic condition. Slightly more GPs than specialists thought it was difficult to find an acceptable doctor (Davidson & Schattner, 2003).

In the UK, a postal survey of GPs and consultants in the South Thames area found in 1999 that although 96% of the doctors were registered with a GP, little use was made of their services. A quarter of GPs were registered within their own practice and 11% looked after members of their own family. Almost a quarter of consultants would bypass their GP to obtain consultant advice. Most doctors prescribed for themselves and their family (Forsythe, Calnan & Wall, 1999). Only 11% of GPs reported availability of occupational health services compared with 95% of consultants, most of whom had never used them for preventive purposes. Presented with illness scenarios affecting themselves, GPs were more likely to self-medicate and go to work than consultants. Within the family, for a child with tonsillitis, GPs were more likely to prescribe an antibiotic but worry less than consultants, and were less likely to call a doctor out or attend at A&E. Perceived barriers were access, confidentiality, lack of occupational health services, and difficulty in finding locum cover for GPs and consequent expense. Overall, the picture presented was of senior doctors with high levels of stress, anxiety, and depression taking very little time off work for illness in general but needing long periods off when they did.

Doctors may deny that they have health problems, and colleagues may collude. Such an approach may run against GMC advice which is that doctors should not rely on their own assessment of risk to patients (Brooke, 1997; General Medical Council, 2001).

Many doctors express the idea that illness is inappropriate for doctors. A 1997 British study interviewed 64 doctors with illness of a month or more and found that cultural values, reinforced by the organisation of medical work, discourage doctors from seeking and obtaining appropriate help when they are ill (McKevitt & Morgan, 1997).

Despite average illness rates, young doctors appear to take less than average sick leave, developing maladaptive patterns such as working when unfit, self-prescribing, and informal rather than formal consultations (Baldwin, Dodd & Wrate, 1997a). The usual response is to go to work and wait and see what happens. Although formal consultations for physical illness are marginally more popular than informal ones, for mental illness the likely response was to see a friend or colleague. A third of this study population of young doctors was not registered with a local GP and most had a poor idea of the role of occupational health.

In a linked study, specific stressors on doctors, e.g. multiple emergency admissions, deaths, and 'menial' tasks, were linked to physical and mental health and performance measures (Baldwin, Dodd & Wrate, 1997b). A feeling of being overwhelmed by work had the biggest impact. This correlated with almost all measures of health outcome, including the number of physical illnesses doctors had had in the last year. The more hours worked, the more likely that the doctors would complain of somatic symptoms.

Guidelines exist for seeking help and advice when ill. In 1995 the BMA produced ethical guidance about doctor-patients and their families (British Medical Association, 1995). They were endorsed by a working party of the Academy of Royal Medical Colleges (Academy of Medical Royal Colleges, 1998) and by the General Medical Council (General Medical Council, 1998).

Why, when they are ill, do doctors behave differently to the general population? There may be many reasons why doctors are reluctant to be perceived to be ill. A qualitative research project using 88 case histories taken from a sample of 1200 Norwegian physicians revealed a pattern of denial and delay in seeking help, despite the occurrence of symptoms that would have suggested diagnoses of concern if they had occurred in patients (Christie & Ingstad, 1996). The doctor who becomes ill has difficulty in admitting the illness. This may be compounded by a role conflict concerning being a patient and a doctor at the same time. The treating physician may also have a role conflict in that he/she is also a colleague. Doctors come to believe that they will not become ill, that doctors should be strong and tough and not overdramatise illness. There is also concern about other people finding out that they are ill, as this may demean them in the eyes of colleagues or patients. This can lead to marked isolation.

Doctors do not make good patients. Part of this is an inability to cede control of care to another. In many cases the doctor-patient knows best. Conversely, sometimes doctors are not allowed to be patients. Doctor colleagues find it difficult to relate to the ill doctor as a patient. There is a difficult balance to be struck. Even when there is a desire to be treated as a patient, healthcare professionals have a tendency to speak to patients in a rather patronising manner and to use language that is inappropriate for someone who is medically trained (Coulter, 1999). The challenge is to use appropriate language and encourage appropriate participation in management decisions whilst not assuming specialist knowledge and ensuring concordance with treatment and advice.

Another explanation is that a non-medical patient is free to construct an explanatory model of illness, whereas a doctor is constrained by his or her knowledge of disease and previous professional experience (Ingstad & Christie, 2001). The doctor's perception of what it is like to be ill is based on the observation of patients who are ill. This can be frightening if previous experience was limited to treating patients with life-threatening illnesses, or frustrating if the previous experience was of patients with chronic disease. It is interesting, although not surprising, that interviews with doctor-patients reveal a common belief that encounters with personal illness strengthened them as doctors.

Assessment of doctors with alleged performance problems

Doctors and dentists assessed by the NCAS routinely undergo an occupational health assessment. It is an holistic assessment comprising an exploration of physical and mental health, workplace and social factors, as well as their relevance to remediation. The context of the assessment is unusual in that referred doctors are not seeking help with health problems and they may wish to hide evidence of illness or of behavioural problems. The doctor concerned can choose how much and what information to disclose. In any clinical assessment, the history is the important component on which diagnoses are based. Examination will confirm the history and facilitate an assessment of the severity of the problem. Occupational health assessments are concerned with not only the existence of medical conditions, but also their impact on fitness to work and on performance at work. Thus, generally speaking, medical examination focuses on the salient features highlighted by the history obtained, with a view to assessing functional capacity.

In some circumstances it is necessary to identify specific health problems, or to exclude their existence. Occupational health assessments sometimes take place because of concerns of poor performance, or in association with disciplinary procedures. The identification of illness might lead to financial penalties or even loss of employment and so this might encourage the individuals to conceal, for example, that they are ill or misusing drugs or alcohol.

The ethics of such assessments are not always straightforward. Whilst knowledge of a doctor's medical condition that might put the health and safety of the public at risk should be disclosed, how far should one go when relatively minor conditions are discovered? Similarly, in the absence of a history of illness, or supporting information to indicate ill health, how far should the screening process be taken?

The choice of any screening tool must satisfy well-established criteria with respect to validity, reliability, accuracy, acceptability and cost-effectiveness. It must be clear why the test is being done and what will happen when the results are obtained. The ethics of managing a case can be considered with recourse to the principles of ethical practice: beneficence, autonomy and confidentiality (Alklint, 2004). One choice is to do nothing, which carries the risk of not dealing with a health problem for which rehabilitation is available or which could lead to further illness. Intervention, on the other hand may highlight a problem, if it exists, but it must be handled carefully and confidentially, on a need to know basis.

Whilst recognising the primacy of protecting patients and the public, an occupational health assessment should not harm doctors who are referred either directly or indirectly, for example as a result of a report sent to the referring Trust. The latter is particularly important because the Trust has no right to gain information about the doctor's health without explicit permission being given beforehand and because, normally, the doctor will return to work in the Trust and could suffer as a result of the information provided. The autonomy of the occupational health service must be emphasised.

The assessment should be evidence-based as far as possible. This is difficult, with respect to physical illnesses, because of the paucity of published information on the subject. Baseline demographic information should include data on birth, current address, address of GP and work address. There should be a training and employment history and a medical history. The referred doctor should be given the opportunity to volunteer information about any symptoms or health concerns, before undertaking a specific review of key symptoms for the main system categories. Specific questions about drug and alcohol intake are essential. In addition, questions about any involvement with the police, or convictions, such as drink driving, can be helpful in building up a picture of social behaviour. A physical examination is required in every case, although it is acknowledged that this is done as an evidence gathering exercise to identify possible illness or exclude markers of disease. This approach can be refined as the evidence base builds up and the findings can be linked to other aspects of the NCAS assessment and the outcomes following the recommendations to the Trusts. A suggested template for assessment is in Appendix A.

Aging and work ability

It is well known that age-related changes occur concerning the functions of specific organs or organ systems (Ilmarinen, 2001). Examples of age-related decline are decreases in cardiorespiratory capacity, muscle strength, hearing acuity and speed of response. From an occupational health perspective, how can the effects of aging on performance be assessed?

In physical jobs 'working capacity' is a term used when assessing fitness for work. In mentally demanding jobs, 'job performance' or a new concept, the 'Work Ability Index' (WAI), might be used to assess the relationship between the resources of individual workers and the demands of their jobs (Ilmarinen, 2001). It is a questionnaire designed to be administered to workers over the age of 45 years, as functional decline can be detected from the age of 30 years, becoming significant around the age of 50 years. However, some workers reach their working peak before the age of 50 years, hence the inclusion of younger workers.

An individual's capacity for work includes:

- health and functional capacities (physical, mental and social)
- education and competence
- values and attitudes
- motivation.

These individual factors are related to work demands (physical and mental), the work community and management and the work environment. The WAI evaluates the interactions of these factors producing a single score to describe the work ability of the individual at a point in time. The WAI questionnaire assesses seven areas:

- current work ability compared to lifetime best
- work ability in relation to the demands of the job
- number of current diseases diagnosed by a physician
- estimated work impairment due to diseases
- sick leave during the past 12 months
- self-assessment of work ability in coming 2 years
- mental resources.

The WAI questionnaire was developed in Finland on a cohort of municipal workers including 61 male and 25 female obstetricians and gynaecologists (Ilmarinen *et al.*, 1991). Job analysis for these physicians determined that the main task was patient care connected with information processing and transmitting, planning the care, arranging the work and negotiating. The work was classified as mental work, rather than physical or mixed work. The main stressors were complex and time-pressured decision making, demands on accuracy in sensory perception, contacts with nurses and colleagues, demands for professional work experience and a need for advanced professional training. Other significant stressors were co-ordination of body movements, stooped and sitting posture, static work – fingers, static work – upper arms, neck and shoulders, and tactile information.

In a longitudinal follow-up study of the cohort of municipal workers, the prevalence of musculo-skeletal diseases increased in the physicians group from 14% to 25% for men and from 14% to 36% for women over a 4-year period (Tuomi, 1991). Similarly, the prevalence of cardiovascular disease increased from 2% to 12% for men, but remained static at 9% for women.

As the mental aspects of work ability are likely to be more prominent in the assessment of physicians, it may be that the WAI is insufficiently sensitive to identify changes in work ability that might affect patient care. Because it relies on self-reporting of changes in work ability, it might be useful when used on reflective practitioners, but not in those who lack insight. Although more work is needed on its use in the UK healthcare sector, there is a possibility that it could be used as a screening tool to identify the need for occupational health interventions in doctors over the age of 45 years.

Factors affecting remediability

Physical illnesses may affect remediability, but this will depend on the nature of the illness and the job for which the doctor is employed. A surgeon with Parkinson's disease may be unable to operate. Multiple sclerosis may lead to performance difficulties, particularly if the physical neurological symptoms are mild but there are cognitive deficits associated with the illness.

Performance may also be impaired by drug treatment. For example, steroid treatment of chronic inflammatory conditions, such as ulcerative colitis or rheumatoid arthritis, may cause both behavioural changes and physical problems. Centrally acting drugs, such as antidepressant medication, may impair performance, as can depression.

Drug and alcohol dependency may militate against remediation, as will impairment of cognitive function.

Physical illness and cognitive impairment

Cognitive impairment is a feature of some physical illnesses including multiple sclerosis, Parkinson's disease, peripheral vascular disease (PVD) and stroke.

In one study 36% patients with Parkinson's disease had evidence of impairment within 2 years of diagnosis (Foltynie *et al.*, 2004).

A recent study of PVD and cognitive function (Waldstein *et al.*, 2003) included patients with stage II peripheral arterial disease (intermittent claudication), stroke, hypertension and normal blood pressure. There was a clear progression. Those with normal blood pressure performed best, with increasing cognitive impairment through the hypertensive patients to the PVD patients and the stroke patients.

Cardiorespiratory fitness may be a predictive factor for preservation of cognitive function (Barnes *et al.*, 2003). A 6-year longitudinal study of non-institutionalised adults aged 55 years and over found that baseline measures of cardiorespiratory fitness were positively correlated with preservation of cognitive function in healthy older adults.

Elevated serum cholesterol in middle age might also be a risk factor for cognitive impairment in later life. A Finnish study of subjects taken from two larger projects (North Karelia Project and FINMONICA – Finnish Multinational Monitoring of Trends and Determinants in Cardiovascular Disease) has shown that high serum cholesterol in mid-life (55–69) increased the risk of cognitive impairment 10 years later. However, cholesterol level or hyperlipidaemia was found to be a factor in other PVD studies (Phillips & MateKole, 1997; Waldstein *et al.*, 2003). Cigarette smoking, based on smoking histories, does not appear to be a risk factor in isolation.

Depression may also cause symptoms of cognitive impairment. Cognitive deficits may be subtle and not detectable using brief screening tests (Foong & Ron, 1998). Self-reported problems with memory or learning may be reliable indicators that formal neuropsychological assessment is merited. Because impairment may be progressive, the identification of cognitively impaired doctors is important with respect to remediation and future fitness to practice.

Asperger's syndrome

Although it is not strictly a mental health problem, some doctors have Asperger's syndrome, a form of autism which is associated with high IQ (Anon, 2004). Such doctors may achieve academic success but difficulty at work. The diagnosis may be delayed, or never made. There is no cure but, with understanding and occupational health support, effective work may be possible.

Symptoms of Asperger's syndrome include:

- Being a loner ill-suited to teamwork.
- Seriousness with an unusual sense of humour.
- Having little or no common sense and lacking 'street credibility'.
- Generating novel and unusual 'off track' solutions to problems.
- A pedantic inflexibility making it difficult to handle all the changes that come with working in the NHS.

- An inability to multiskill, so that working in acute specialties is disastrous.
- Subtle speech difficulties, making communication with colleagues and patients problematic.
- Eccentricities – 'the mad professor' – making it hard to fit into conformist medicine.

Should doctors have routine health screens?

Suggestions of carrying out health screens on employees are made frequently in occupational health practice. There is a general belief that this ought to be a good thing, as it will lead to the early identification of disease and subsequent treatment. It is desirable, therefore, as a form of secondary prevention. However, most clinical screening tools do not make good community screening tools as they are not sufficiently sensitive or specific when the likelihood of finding a disease is low. Thus they are not cost-effective or efficient and they can create unnecessary anxiety in individual people as a result of a false positive result.

Most health assessments in the NHS are questionnaire-based, requiring doctors to declare health problems at the start of a new job. Doctors who work for the same employer for many years might not have an additional health assessment, unless they develop an illness that requires time off work or they volunteer that they have a problem.

However, it can be argued that doctors have jobs that require high-level performance. Failure may have adverse effects on the health and safety of the public in general and of the vulnerable members of society in particular. Doctors work long hours and are known to suffer from psychiatric illnesses and to misuse drugs and alcohol. This is compounded by the fact that they do not take their own health seriously and they rarely consult their general practitioner, if they have one.

Doctors are often compared with airline pilots, who undergo routine medical assessments (MacDonald, 2002). It is suggested that junior doctors work in an environment which is 'psychotoxic', yet they do not enjoy the support that is given to pilots in the form of regular evaluation and health checks coupled with better working conditions. To meet their medical standards, pilots must have excellent distance vision and good near and intermediate vision. Hearing standards must be met and there must be cardiovascular fitness. Other conditions that might affect pilots include asthma, renal calculi, chronic organ failures, and severe mental illness, such as psychotic illness or bipolar disorders (see www.leftseat.com/FAAforms.htm and www.caa.co.uk/srg/med/default.asp?page=539). Pilots usually work in teams and so the occurrence of a debilitating illness should not be catastrophic, although it would increase the risk to the public. Doctors also work in safety-critical jobs, often in teams but also as individual practitioners.

Routine medical checks for doctors involved in critical care jobs would be a sensible precaution to ensure fitness to practise, with the offer of support if necessary. They might be particularly important for doctors aged 45 years or more. In light of the high prevalence of psychological distress amongst healthcare workers, including doctors, the use of a screening questionnaire, such as the General Health questionnaire, could be considered. Evidence of hypertension, cardiac disease or peripheral vascular disease should be sought with respect to risk factors for cognitive impairment. Routine 'well person' checks such as body mass index, blood pressure and ECG and urinalysis for sugar could be implemented, along with screening of hearing and vision. In annual air crew medicals for Royal Navy pilots, a medical review of preliminary screening data strongly predicts the outcome of the medical with respect to fitness to fly (Roberts, 2003). The preliminary screening tests are height, weight, urinalysis, blood pressure and visual acuity in all cases and audiometry, Harvard step tests score, lung function, ECG and lifestyle questions in some cases. The preliminary data and the opinion of the pilot that he/she wished to see a doctor were both strong predictors of a positive finding (abnormal finding) at the medical assessment. Of the preliminary parameters tested, body mass index and urinalysis were significant predictors of positive outcomes at medical assessment. Routine screening should be part of a more comprehensive assessment of performance, including job-specific tests of capability and 360-degree appraisal.

Areas for future research

There is a need for greater intelligence about the prevalence of physical illness in doctors and about how this impacts on fitness for work. Qualitative studies exploring the effects of illness on performance as well as attitudes to managing illness could be illuminating. Research into the effects on performance of chronic illnesses such as diabetes, epilepsy and inflammatory conditions is needed, looking at both the illness and the effects of treatment.

More information is needed about the prevalence of alcohol misuse in the medical profession and factors that cause and or sustain it. In addition, research into cannabis abuse is required, particularly amongst junior doctors, to assess whether this is likely to have a significant effect on patient care. Attitudes to drug and alcohol testing, linked to treatment and rehabilitation programmes, should be explored.

More research is necessary to improve our understanding of cognitive impairment: its relevance to clinical practice and methods of assessment in physical illness. It seems likely that reliance on just one testing modality will be insufficient. A combination of neuropsychological testing and imaging seems to be a way forward but is not practical in routine clinical assessments. The development of a clinical screening tool would be advantageous. Tests of executive function and verbal performance seem to hold most promise. The screening test would have to be easy to carry out in a consulting room and not take too long to complete.

Appendix A: Occupational health assessment of doctors referred to the NCAS

Clinical notes

Name		DoB:
Address		

Phone		Email	
Job		Employer	

NCAS number	
NCAS casework manager	
Specific questions	
Assessor	
Date of assessment	
Duration of assessment	

Training and employment:

Any health complaints:

Past medical history:

Systematic enquiry: (enter Nil if no evidence of problem)

Depression

Anxiety

Alcohol

Drugs

Neurological

Musculo-skeletal

Cardiorespiratory

Forensic (e.g. drink-driving conviction or other involvement with the police)

Social

Beliefs: (work-relatedness)

Examination: Declined

Mental health screening tools:

Type	Score	Reference	Comment

Vision: Distance: Near: Intermediate:
Hearing: Conversation: Rinne/Weber:
Urinalysis:
Height: Weight: BMI:
Drug/alcohol screen:
Physical:

Conclusions (with reasons):
Fit for further assessment

Any health problems

Could the health problems have affected performance?

Are any of the following tests required?:
Cognitive impairment

Personality

Motor-coordination

The physical assessment

In addition to general observation for signs of illness, blood pressure should be taken and assessment of the radial pulse and auscultation of the heart carried out. Examination of the respiratory system and abdomen will complete the assessment for possible cardiorespiratory disease and for signs of chronic liver disease. There should be a functional assessment of the musculo-skeletal system to assess the range of movement of all the major joints and spine. Similarly, an assessment of the nervous system should assess the presence of muscle weakness, inco-ordination and ataxia and tremor. Fundoscopy can ensure that there are no lens or retinal problems. Visual acuity should be measured to assess distance vision and near vision. This can be performed by any appropriate means, such as the use of Snellen charts, or by using screening equipment, such as a Keystone vision screener, which is used widely by occupational health departments. The finding of monocular vision is not usually clinically relevant, although it may be if the referred doctor is required to carry out microsurgery or stereotactic surgery (Poole *et al.*, 2002). Consideration should be given to testing colour vision.

A simple test of hearing can be carried out by adopting a quiet conversational tone during the consultation and, perhaps, covering the examiner's mouth. If a doctor volunteers a hearing difficulty then the usual clinical tests using a tuning fork are carried out after examination of the ears. If a hearing loss is identified, referral for audiometry should be considered.

Routine urinalysis for blood sugar and protein in the absence of symptoms is not usually a useful screening tool. However, at this stage in the development of the health assessment it is probably worth including, particularly for doctors aged 45 years or over.

References

Academy of Medical Royal Colleges (1998) *Report of a Working Party*. AMRC, London.

Alklint T (2004) Alcohol abuse in the workplace: some ethical considerations. In: P Westerholm *et al*. (eds) *Practical Ethics*. Radcliffe Medical Press, Oxford, pp. 167–76.

Anon (2004) Life as a doctor with Asperger's Syndrome. *BMJ Careers*. **329**: 130.

Baldwin PJ, Dodd M and Wrate RW (1997a) Young doctors' health 2. Health and health behaviour. *Social Science and Medicine*. **45**(1): 41–4.

Baldwin PJ, Dodd M and Wrate RW (1997b) Young doctors' health 1: How do working conditions affect attitudes, health and performance? *Social Science and Medicine*. **45**(1): 35–40.

Barnes DE *et al*. (2003) A longitudinal study of cardiorespiratory fitness and cognitive function in healthy older adults. *Journal of the American Geriatrics Society*. **51**(4): 459–65.

Boisaubin EV and Levine RE (2001) Identifying and assisting the impaired physician. *American Journal of Medical Science*. **322**(1): 31–6.

British Medical Association (1997) *Meeting the Needs of Doctors with Disabilities*. British Medical Association, London.

British Medical Association (1995) *Ethical Responsibilities Involved in Treating Doctor-patients*. British Medical Association, London.

Brooke D (1997) Ethical debate – why are doctors ambivalent about patients who misuse alcohol? Doctors neglect their own alcohol problems as well as those of their patients. *BMJ*. **315**(7118): 1299.

Bruguera M *et al*. (2001) Care of doctors to their health care – results of a postal survey. *Medicina Clinica*. **117**(13): 492–4.

Carpenter LM, Swerdlow AJ and Fear NT (1997) Mortality of doctors in different specialties: findings from a cohort of 20 000 NHS consultants. *Occupational & Environmental Medicine*. **54**(6): 388–95.

Christie V and Ingstad B (1996) Reluctant to be perceived to be ill – the case of the physician. In: O Larsen (ed.) *The Shaping of a Profession: physicians in Norway past and present*. Science History Publications, Canton, MA, pp. 491–9.

Coulter A (1999) Paternalism or partnership? *BMJ*. **319**: 719–20.

Davidson SK and Schattner PL (2003) Doctors' health-seeking behaviour: a questionnaire survey. *Medical Journal of Australia*. **179**(6): 302–5.

Department of Health (2000) *Hepatitis B Infected Health Care Workers: guidance on implementation of Health Service Circular 2000/020*. Department of Health, London.

Doll R *et al*. (1994a) Mortality in relation to smoking: 40 years' observations on male British doctors. *BMJ*. **309**(6959): 901–11.

Doll R *et al*. (1994b) Mortality in relation to consumption of alcohol: 13 years' observations on male British doctors. *BMJ*. **309**(6959): 911–18.

Emmett EA (1987) *Health Problems of Health Care Workers*. Hanley & Belfus Inc., Philadelphia, PA.

Foltynie T *et al*. (2004) The cognitive ability of an incident cohort of Parkinson's patients in the UK. The CamPaIGN study. *Brain*. **127**(3): 550–60.

Foong J and Ron M (1998) Multiple sclerosis and other neurological disorders. *Current Opinion in Psychiatry*. **11**(3): 311–14.

Forsythe M, Calnan M and Wall B (1999) Doctors as patients: postal survey examining consultants' and general practitioners' adherence to guidelines. *BMJ*. **319**(7210): 605–8.

General Medical Council (2001) *Good Medical Practice* [online] (3e). General Medical Council, London. Available at: www.gmc-uk.org/standards/default.htm [Accessed 22 September 2004].

General Medical Council (1998) Doctors should not treat themselves or their families [online]. *GMC News*. **3**(Summer). Available at: www.gmc-uk.org/news/gmcnews/gmcnews3.htm#self-medication [Accessed 25 October 2004].

Harrison J and Redfern N (2001) Flexible training scheme for doctors who are ill. *BMJ*. **322**(7296): S2.

Hirst R (2003) Life as a doctor with diabetes. *BMJ*. **327**(7427): S181.

Ilmarinen JE (2001) Aging Workers. *Occupational & Environmental Medicine*. **58**(8): 546–52.

Ilmarinen J et al. (1991) Background and objectives of Finnish research-project on aging workers in municipal occupations. *Scandinavian Journal of Work Environment & Health*. **17**(Suppl 1): 7–11.

Ingstad B and Christie VM (2001) Encounters with illness: the perspective of the sick doctor. *Anthropology and Medicine*. **8**(2/3): 201–10.

Litchfield P (ed.) (1995) *Health Risks to the Health Care Professional*. Royal College of Physicians of London in association with the Faculty of Occupational Medicine, London.

MacDonald E (2002) One pilot son, one medical son. *BMJ*. **324**(7345): 1105.

Marsden C (2000) Akinetic-rigid syndromes. In: JGG Ledingham and DA Warrell (eds) *Concise Oxford Textbook of Medicine*. Oxford University Press, Oxford, chs. 13 and 20.

McKevitt C and Morgan M (1997) Illness doesn't belong to us. *Journal of the Royal Society of Medicine*. **90**(9): 491–5.

Parker G and Kalucy M (1999) Depression comorbid with physical illness. *Current Opinion in Psychiatry*. **12**(1): 87–92.

Pattani S, Constantinovici N and Williams S (2001) Who retires early from the NHS because of ill health and what does it cost? A national cross sectional study. *BMJ*. **322**(7280): 208–9.

Phillips NA and MateKole CC (1997) Cognitive deficits in peripheral vascular disease – a comparison of mild stroke patients and normal control subjects. *Stroke*. **28**(4): 777–84.

Poole CJ et al. (2002) Guidance on standards of health for clinical care workers. *Occupational Medicine*. **52**(1): 17–24.

Poole CJ et al. (1997) Deficient colour vision and interpretation of histopathology slides: cross sectional study. *BMJ*. **315**(7118): 1279–81.

Pullen D et al. (1995) Medical care of doctors. *Medical Journal of Australia*. **162**(9): 481–4.

Richards JG (1999) The health and health practices of doctors and their families. *New Zealand Medical Journal*. **112**(1084): 96–9.

Roberts A (2003) Can the design of the annual aircrew medical be improved? (Dissertation for MFOM.)

Stanton J and Caan W (2003) How many doctors are sick? *BMJ*. **326**(7391): S97.

Tuomi K et al. (1991) Prevalence and incidence rates of diseases and work ability in different work categories of municipal occupations. *Scandinavian Journal of Work Enviironment & Health*. **17**(Suppl 1): 67–74.

Waldstein SR et al. (2003) Peripheral arterial disease and cognitive function. *Psychosomatic Medicine*. **65**(5): 757–63.

Williams S, Michie S and Pattani S (1998) *Improving the Health of the NHS Workforce: report of the partnership on the health of the NHS workforce*. The Nuffield Trust, London.

Chapter 2

A perspective on stress and depression

Jenny Firth-Cozens

Mental health problems in doctors have been the focus of researchers' attention for decades, with good longitudinal studies allowing us to consider their long-term predictors, in particular of general occupational stress, depression and substance abuse. The focus on these areas is not arbitrary, as findings show that doctors suffer from elevated levels in each, compared to the general public or to other professional groups (Firth-Cozens, 1999b; Ghodse, 2000), while other psychiatric conditions such as psychosis and personality disorders are likely to occur in similar proportions to any other population. This chapter focuses primarily on studies of stress and depression since they are highly related, though the frequent comorbidity between depression and alcohol use will also be discussed where appropriate. Substance abuse in general is the focus of Chapter 3.

The chapter looks at the levels of stress and depression in doctors and their effects upon patient care, discusses their individual and organisational causes, and finally outlines interventions to reduce the problem.

Levels of stress and depression in doctors

Reported levels of stress in health service professionals – especially in doctors and nurses – are higher than those in British workers as a whole, with around 28% showing above-threshold symptoms at any one time (Wall *et al.*, 1997). This study and others which measure stress use instruments that provide indications of general psychiatric morbidity in a population; for example, the General Health Questionnaire (GHQ), a well-validated measure of stress (Goldberg, 1978) which is particularly useful in judging levels of psychiatric morbidity in the community, but which has also been shown to be a reliable measure of work-related stress in a population. Where measures of depression rather than stress are used, studies show the prevalence of depression in UK doctors to be of the order of 10–20% (Ghodse, 2000), similar to the United States: current US estimates are that approximately 15% of physicians are impaired through depression or substance misuse at some point in their careers (Boisaubin & Levine, 2001).

Figure 2.1 describes the findings of a UK longitudinal study (Firth-Cozens, 2004) where both stress and depression have been considered in a group of medical students (n=314) who became general practitioners and hospital doctors. These data support the general findings described above which show that stress is a larger problem than depression in doctors, but both behave similarly; in fact in this study the relationship between the two is around r=0.7 on each assessment. The first column shows the percentage of British workers above threshold on the 12-item version of the GHQ. This is compared with the last four columns, which show the cohort of doctors followed over 17 years from 1983 when they were fourth year medical students to 2000 when they were senior doctors aged around 40 years. The graph shows remarkable consistency with around 30% indicating above-threshold stress at all times apart from their first postgraduate year, when it was much higher. In fact, some of the problems of that year have been relieved by various policy changes, particularly around establishing legal maximum hours of work, and more recent studies of house officers (HOs) usually show much lower levels (Kapur, Borrill & Stride, 1998), though these vary considerably depending on the hospital or the type of rotation undertaken (Firth-Cozens *et al.*, 2000).

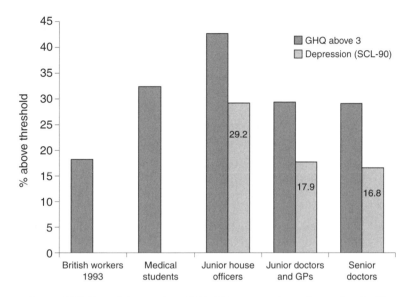

Figure 2.1 Stress (GHQ) and depression (SCL-90): proportions above threshold.

The grey columns of the final three assessments show depression levels on those occasions (using the depression scale from the Symptom Check List-90 (Derogatis *et al.*, 1973)). Again it can be seen that, after the first postgraduate year, levels stay at around 17%. Again, the high levels for HOs in 1985 may at least in part have been due to very long work hours, which are known to lower mood (Weinger & Ancoli-Israel, 2002). While the GHQ has been widely used around the world as an indicator of general stress and potential psychiatric morbidity and so allows useful comparisons, depression is measured by a wide array of assessments, some of which are discussed later. Perhaps because of this variation, some studies have found considerably higher levels of depression in doctors, especially in general practitioners, using different measures (Caplan, 1994). Depression has also been demonstrated by the finding that suicide is a disproportionately high cause of death in doctors (Center *et al.*, 2003), particularly so in women, both in the UK (Hawton *et al.*, 2001) and elsewhere (Hem, 2004).

Gender differences

Although gender differences in doctors' stress levels are rarely found, women doctors have higher levels of depression, and, as Table 2.1 (Firth-Cozens, 2004) suggests, this is due to significantly elevated levels in female hospital doctors. These differences do not appear until graduation, and are not predicted by student levels of depression, as is the case for male doctors (Brewin & Firth-Cozens, 1997). It is likely, therefore, that female doctors' elevated depression levels are more to do with the workplace – in particular, the hospital setting – while men's are more likely to be dispositional.

Table 2.1 SCL-D depression mean item scores for senior male and female general practitioners and hospital doctors (Firth-Cozens, 2004)

	Men	*Women*
General practitioners	.80	.83
Hospital doctors	.62	1.12

Co-morbidity

There is considerable co-morbidity between depression, suicide, alcoholism and drug abuse. A study of 100 recovered alcoholic women doctors (Bissell & Skorina, 1987) found that 73 had serious suicidal ideation prior to becoming sober, and more than half of these made at least one suicide attempt. In fact, this psychiatric co-morbidity in doctors appears to be growing (Angres *et al.*, 2003) or perhaps is just better recognised. Alcoholism has been recognised as a particular problem for doctors over many years whether it is measured by psychiatric admissions or by cirrhotic deaths (Harrison & Chick, 1994). It is also a largely hidden problem, with doctors taking many years to admit to addiction (Brooke, Edwards & Taylor, 1991) and their colleagues being slow to confront it (Sclare, 1979). Unlike other professions, alcohol problems in doctors have been reported to increase with age in the US. In particular, women medical students' level of alcohol use rises over their training till it equals that of male colleagues on graduation (Flaherty & Richman, 1993), whereas most students drink less as they progress.

As the levels of drug addiction, particularly opiates, rises in the UK and elsewhere, it is very likely that this is also increasing in doctors: levels of use amongst UK house officers are reportedly high (Birch, Ashton & Kamali, 1998); a European study found that psychoactive drug use in medical doctors was higher than that in the general population (Domenighetti *et al.*, 1991); and in Australia one State programme for impaired doctors reported 45% of referrals for drug misuse and 7% for alcohol (Farmer, 2002). In addition, since doctors who are addicted usually misappropriate their drugs from the workplace, this creates a particular problem for health services (Strang, 1998).

Doctors are also likely to have similar rates of other psychiatric illnesses to other groups; thus a small proportion is likely to suffer from schizophrenia, manic depression, post-traumatic stress disorder (Firth-Cozens, Midgley & Burges, 1999) and eating or personality disorders, with the 'rogue doctor' probably coming within the last group (Crow *et al.*, 2003). There is little evidence about their prevalence, or about the extent to which they are recognised and dealt with by colleagues. In addition, doctors who have a serious physical health problem may, like most people, also experience depression (*see* Chapter 1), as may those who are suffering from cognitive problems (*see* Chapter 4).

The effects of mental health problems on patient care

These disorders have a fundamental effect on the doctors, their families (Dumelow, Littlejohns & Griffiths, 2000), and on the quality of service provided (Firth-Cozens, 2001). Doctors are under-treated for depression themselves (Lindeman *et al.*, 1999) and under-treat depression in their patients too (Simon & VonKorff, 1995; Pirkis & Burgess, 1998). It is likely that this applies to alcohol problems as well. Evidence shows that healthy habits in a general practitioner lead to greater prevention-related counselling of patients (Frank *et al.*, 2000): if you are in denial about your own problems, you may be less likely to recognise them in patients too, putting them at risk as well as yourself.

The effects of stress, depression and alcohol use on patient care have been described in a number of reviews (Firth-Cozens, 2001). In particular, excessive alcohol use affects most organs of the body, but has definite effects upon the functioning of the brain, some of which can be long-lasting (*see* Chapter 3). Less is known about the long-term use of illegal drugs, though even cannabis raises the likelihood of later psychosis (Henquet *et al.*, 2005), and their illegality in itself can create problems for patient care.

Although most studies of the effects of psychological symptoms on performance relate only to stress levels, it is likely that they will apply equally to the effects of depression. In both depression and high stress, people suffer from memory, concentration and attention loss, find it difficult to make decisions and often become very irritable. All these cognitive and mood effects will inevitably affect the quality of doctoring given. For example, studies have shown that irritability and anger with patients is a feature of doctors' stress (Firth-Cozens & Greenhalgh, 1997) and, in a study which followed house officers prior to and eight weeks after beginning their first jobs, stress levels and error-making rose in relation to each other (Houston & Allt, 1997). In another study, doctors who had shown high stress levels on two consecutive assessments were compared with those who had been below threshold at both times, and the 'always stressed' group reported making significantly more mistakes than the 'never stressed' group. This is likely to indicate that high stress results in more error; however, in addition, the first group was significantly more self-critical, and it may be that they were perceiving more adverse events to have been caused by them (Firth-Cozens & Morrison, 1989).

High levels of stress have been linked to cognitive failures (Reason, 1988), which in turn may negatively affect patient care. For example, Parkes (Broadbent *et al.*, 1982) found a highly significant relationship between cognitive failures and stress scores in nurses who had worked on high-stress wards. No such relationship was present on low-stress wards. Other studies link low job satisfaction (always highly related to high stress symptoms) to lower patient satisfaction, higher no-show rates and lower compliance in patients (Linn *et al.*, 1995; DiMatteo *et al.*, 1993).

Finally, a study by Jones *et al.* (1988) has shown that medication errors in hospitals are related to staff stress scores. Moreover, when they designed an intervention for stress management and compared 22 hospitals which had the intervention with controls (22 others matched for urban/rural, beds and previous litigation claims), they found that the intervention group's malpractice claims dropped from 31 to 9, while the control groups remained virtually identical. This demonstrates well the links between stress and performance, but also that successful interventions will reduce the former and raise the latter.

In addition to the effects on patient care and on the doctors themselves, these mental health problems are expensive to organisations in terms of sickness absence, suspensions, litigation and early retirement. The most common reason for a doctor taking early retirement from the NHS is psychiatric (Pattani, Constantinovici & Williams, 2001). Because the direct and indirect effects of stress and depression on patient care are manifestly significant, the causes for these problems need to be understood so that remedies can be put in place.

The individual and organisational causes of stress and depression in doctors

There has been a considerable debate over the last two decades about the relative importance of individual factors and occupational or life factors in terms of predicting stress and depression, but evidence shows that both will play a role. For example, depressed students who become psychiatrists are likely to remain depressed, stressed and dissatisfied 17 years later; on the other hand, depressed students who become pathologists have much lower levels of subsequent stress and higher job satisfaction (Firth-Cozens, Lema & Firth, 1999). Despite similar levels of initial depression, one group has made a career choice which gets them particularly close to patients who may have similar problems, and they are not helped by this; while the other group has chosen to work as separately as possible from patients, which has been beneficial in some respects. It seems from this that some work conditions can go some way towards alleviating the experience of stress. This literature, on person-job fit, has rarely been considered in medicine.

This section considers the principal individual and organisational causes of stress found in the literature. Since stress, depression and alcohol use are likely to have a number of highly related causes, and since co-morbidity is such a feature of their presentation, the literature reported under this section principally refers to 'stress' unless the evidence indicates differences for other conditions.

Individual causes

Life events

Stress and depression are strongly linked to life events, especially those concerning loss, and these are probably summative in their effects (Turner & Lloyd, 2004). Young doctors in particular often suffer from a number of life events (moving jobs and houses frequently, relationship problems, marriages, new babies and young children, for example) and some of these will come together over the early years of their careers.

Gender

As we mentioned above, women hospital doctors are an at-risk group for depression, particularly if they are working full-time and have children (Firth-Cozens & Bonanno, 1999). Unlike their male colleagues, differences in symptoms do not appear when they are students but only in the first postgraduate year, and so are likely to be more job-related than in men (Brewin & Firth-Cozens, 1997). A large

Norwegian study (Tyssen *et al.*, 2004) of suicidal planning in doctors found that its predictors were: being female, living alone, sick leave due to depression, and subjective health complaints.

Alcohol

Alcohol problems may well begin early, both in men and in women (Brooke, Edwards & Taylor, 1991), and this too may contribute to the higher than usual levels of suicide, particularly in female doctors. A longitudinal study of doctors in Sweden has found that frequent overtime worked 24 years earlier was associated with heavy alcohol use among women (Michelsen & Bildt, 2003). This may link to the finding that women hospital doctors are most at risk for depression.

Coping strategies

A number of studies have shown that particular ways of coping with adverse events are predictive of stress and depression (Firth-Cozens & Morrison, 1989; Koeske, Kirk & Koeske, 1993; Tattersall, Bennet & Pugh, 1999). If work-related incidents are coped with by avoidance, dismissal or denial, people are more likely to suffer higher symptom levels. The other poor method of coping is through alcohol or drug use and this is highly linked to depression (Holahan *et al.*, 2004). That young doctors use alcohol to cope with difficult work situations is illustrated by the following quotation from a longitudinal study (Firth-Cozens, 2004):

> 'I am so tired so often that I just want to collapse in a chair and have a few drinks. This causes shaky hands the next day so epidurals etc are more difficult.'

Some will learn early that alcohol or drugs seem to be an effective way to cope with the stressors of the day (albeit in the short term), while the time demands of their training provide them with no real opportunities to learn other ways of relieving these.

Personality

Studies of the effects of personality upon mental health and job-related behaviours ideally need to be longitudinal. Although good longitudinal studies exist in this field, whatever personality factors the researchers chose to measure in the first assessment, and which proved to be predictive, are those that stay for the life of the study. This means that there may be many other personality factors which have not been assessed in this way but which may also be important in terms of their predictive power.

Longitudinal studies outside medicine have isolated a number of personality factors which may have long-term implications for health-risk behaviours such as alcohol dependence (Caspi *et al.*, 1997), and these may have implications for medicine (*see* Chapter 5). In terms of the job interacting with personality, longitudinal studies of alcohol use in medicine have shown that being humiliated as a young doctor and having a vulnerable personality are predictive of later substance abuse (Richman, 1992).

In the longitudinal study of doctors referred to above (Firth-Cozens, 2004), self-criticism measured as students has proved to be an important predictor of depression over a number of years, particularly for men (Brewin & Firth-Cozens, 1997; Firth-Cozens, 1992). This depression is 'characterized by self-criticism and feelings of unworthiness, inferiority, failure, and guilt. These individuals engage in constant harsh self-scrutiny and evaluation and have a chronic fear of being disapproved of and criticized ... They strive for excessive achievement and perfection, are often highly competitive and work hard ...' (Blatt & Zuroff, 1992). As is described in Chapter 5, the fear of being criticised may make feedback difficult with these people: although they may privately always look to themselves for the first cause of blame, they may still find it difficult to take blame from others. If they are particularly defensive they may have interpersonal difficulties along with depression.

However, being particularly *low* in self-criticism (blaming others), while apparently good for one's own mental health (Firth-Cozens & Morrison, 1989), is not ideal for one's relationships, and is related to more interpersonal difficulties with colleagues and patients than is being *high* in self-criticism (Firth-Cozens, 1995). The main predictors of young doctors having problems with their seniors is that they had lower self-criticism measured as students, and at that time reported their fathers to be older, more strict, powerful and hard-to-please (Firth-Cozens, 1992). Perhaps being loath to consider one's own responsibility in events, even to oneself, may be a defence against the acts of early authoritarian figures.

Early experience

A number of longitudinal studies have shown the importance of early experience on doctors' mental health (Firth-Cozens, 1992; Vaillant, Sobowale & McArthur, 1972; Thomas & Duszynski, 1974). For example, one study has found that the main predictor of depression in general practitioners was sibling rivalry when young, and the main stressor for them now was the feeling that workload was unfairly shared (Firth-Cozens, 1998). A doctor who enters general practice to recreate and repair early family relationships may be disappointed by the inevitable inequalities which can be perceived depending on which way the cake is cut. Although the early experiences of doctors are unchangeable, an understanding of how they may interact with the workplace is useful in terms of remediation.

Of all the psychoanalytical theorists, Kohut places most emphasis on work as being an integral part of mental health. His self-psychology (Kohut, 1971) is useful in beginning to understand the two groups of doctors discussed above – those with high or low self-criticism. In his work the 'self' is a system which constantly compensates for early attacks in its struggle to achieve equilibrium and mental health. Parental figures may or may not show appropriate empathic responses to the young infant's exhibitionistic efforts, and normal or pathological development respectively may follow from this. The good parent mirrors the infant's attempts to be creative or achieving, and it is this mirroring which becomes internalised in the healthy child and later in the adult's ambition and pleasure at work. As I have suggested elsewhere (Firth-Cozens, 1997), if someone has insufficient or inappropriate mirroring when young – and children of professional parents and especially doctors (Gerber, 1983) may get less than most, simply because of a lack of time – they are likely to use their work to get the appreciation they need, but will remain self-critical.

However, if they are particularly damaged, Kohut suggests they may create a grandiose defence system which projects worthlessness onto others; that is, they are unusually *low* in self-criticism and will blame other people. This grandiosity, arrogance and even hostility may actually be rewarded in some cultures, at least in the short term (Van Kleef, De Dreu & Manstead, 2004), though as it becomes less appropriate within medicine, disciplinary bodies may see more of these doctors.

Once doctors have left the training grades, they have few superiors to provide the mirroring they may still want and, in a competitive culture such as medicine, colleagues may be less than forthcoming with praise. Some specialties, such as surgery (which consistently has the lowest stress and depression scores in all studies (Firth-Cozens, Lema & Firth, 1999), still have reasonable appreciation from patients, while others have very little – particularly psychiatry, which consistently has the highest stress and depression scores. Feelings of failure at work often precipitate depression (Czander, 1993), and in the growing culture of complaints and litigation these may be increasingly difficult to avoid (Vincent, 1996).

Organisational causes

Organisations can undoubtedly have a very great effect upon the stress levels of their staff. In a large national survey of NHS Trusts (Wall *et al.*, 1997) the percentages of those above threshold on the GHQ varied between Trusts from 17% (below the general working population) to 33% (considerably above it). Similarly, in a study of stress levels in pre-registration house officers in London hospitals (Firth-Cozens *et al.*, 2000), mean GHQ scores in the various organisations varied from 8.1 to 15.3. This had nothing to do with the size of the hospital, and was most likely to be due to their culture and management. It is clear from these studies that organisations have a major effect on staff health.

This was also the finding of a study which compared 64 doctors, nurses and ancillary workers with high scores (>4) on the GHQ *and* a depressive or anxiety disorder confirmed by clinical interview, with 64 staff with low GHQ scores (Weinberg & Creed, 2000). It found that the two groups worked similar hours and had similar responsibility; however, those who had a high GHQ score and a disorder had a greater number of objective stressful situations both in and out of work, and more objective work problems. Even after the effects of personal vulnerability to psychiatric disorders and ongoing social stress outside work were taken into account, stressful situations at work contributed to their anxiety and depressive disorders. The most striking difference between the groups was a lack of support from their manager in those with disorders. Similarly in the Whitehall II study (North *et al.*, 1996), support from supervisors and colleagues reduced the chances of poor mental health and sickness absence.

Leaders and teamwork

Leaders, whether of teams or organisations, have been shown by meta-analytic studies to be a key source of stress for staff (*see* Chapter 9). In addition, the functioning of the team itself has dramatic effects upon the mental health of at least some of its members (*see* Chapter 8). Studies of health workers in general (Carter & West, 1999) and of pre-registration house officers (Firth-Cozens, 1999a) show that those in effective teams (with clearly defined roles, recognised externally as a functional team, whose members work together to achieve them, with different roles for different members) have lower stress levels than those in teams which do not meet these criteria. In addition, the study of house officers shows that those who *know* they are in a multidisciplinary team have significantly lower stress levels, feel more supported, and think their skills are being used better than those who do not realise they are in multidisciplinary teams. Clearly, if you recognise the breadth of your team you have more people to go to for support and, as house officers, feel that your skills are more valued than if you see yourself simply at the bottom of a medical hierarchy.

Control

A factor consistently found to be a stressor in organisations in general is having low discretion or control over how the job is carried out (Payne and Firth-Cozens, 1987). Although this is less of a problem in medicine, general practitioners in particular see the control they have enjoyed over their working lives as being gradually eroded by policy changes, and this is a major factor in their intentions for early retirement, which in turn impinges upon patient care (Newton *et al.*, 2004).

Overload and resources

Workload is dealt with fully in Chapter 10. Its relationship to stress levels is usually complex and not always apparent in medicine (Baldwin, Dodd & Wrate, 1997). Nevertheless, the finding that frequent overtime relates to heavy alcohol use in women 24 years later (Michelsen & Bildt, 2003) is disturbing. It may be that cross-sectional studies or brief longitudinal studies simply cannot capture these long-term effects. In addition, the tiredness that may follow long hours lowers mood and this can make other aspects of the job, such as a complaint or the death of a child, more difficult to endure.

What is usually overlooked in research is the effect of a lack of resources on overload and stress levels: if dependable staff with whom you are used to working are not available in adequate numbers, if equipment is poor or absent, if the workload is so unremitting that there is less time for proper communication or support, then stress levels will undoubtedly rise and patient care will deteriorate. Although not fully tested, evidence for this commonsense hypothesis is emerging from the safety literature (Carthey *et al.*, 2003; Roberts, 1990).

Stressors in medicine

The factors mentioned above are universal in their potential effects, but there are also stressors peculiar to medicine. These are likely to differ at different times and at different points throughout a career, and also by the way they are measured. For example, using the Sources of Stress Questionnaire (created from previous literature and findings to quantitatively assess the perceived levels and frequency of particular named stressors) it was found that relationships with senior doctors were a major issue (Firth-Cozens, 1995). However, asking the same young doctors to write about a recent stressful incident brought out primarily descriptions of patients' death or suffering. More recently, senior doctors report that their sources of stress involve the growing expectations of patients, fears about making mistakes, and the increase in litigation and complaints (Vincent, 1996).

Whereas sleep loss has regularly been implicated in the lowering of mood in doctors (Weinger & Ancoli-Israel, 2002) (*see* Chapter 10) and often of performance, this is likely to be considerably reduced as a problem with the introduction of the European Working Time Directive. However, teams will still have a role in considering the implications in terms of patient safety of the work performance of any staff who are sleep-deprived from any cause.

Assessment

If there are any symptoms suggesting psychological distress, including irritability or bad behaviour which is uncharacteristic, then specialist assessment is recommended. Clinical assessment is always preferable, though there are also a number of questionnaire measures which the assessor may use. These should, of course, only be given and interpreted by qualified people.

Within a population, such as a department or a Trust, psychological distress or potential psychiatric morbidity can be assessed well using the General Health Questionnaire 12-item measure (Goldberg, 1978). However, this provides only a snapshot of symptom levels at the time for any particular individual, and is not recommended as a change measure. A simple test of depression and anxiety is the Hospital Anxiety and Depression Scale (HADS (Dunbar *et al.*, 2000)), while a good measure of psychiatric symptoms and change is the SCL-90 (Derogatis, Lipman & Covi, 1973), which also provides scales and profiles for particular diagnoses such as depression, obsessional-compulsive disorders, etc. For alcohol assessment, the AUDIT tool was developed as a screening test for detecting harmful and hazardous drinking in generalist settings like primary care or general hospitals (Saunders *et al.*, 1993; Heather & Kaner, 2003).

Remediation

Figure 2.2 demonstrates a systems approach to the causes of poor patient care (Firth-Cozens, 2001). It shows that there are direct and indirect latent and active organisational influences on care, and some of these involve known stressors for doctors. Doctors in turn have various individual factors, such as personality and levels of competence, which again may directly affect patient care (for example, by poor communication or misdiagnosis) or indirectly by leading to their own stress, depression or alcohol abuse, which in turn will affect patient care directly, and also be affected by any litigation or complaints which follow.

However, the model also shows that interventions can take place at many points in the system. At the organisational level, interventions can take place to improve management practices and create an open and fair organisational culture (*see* Chapter 7), improving leadership and teamwork skills (*see* Chapters 9 and 8) and changing attitudes to safety (Helmreich & Willhelm, 1991).

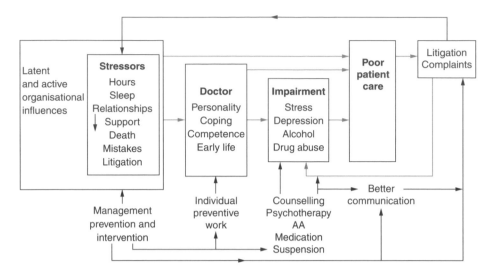

Figure 2.2 A systems approach to the causes of poor patient care.

Organisational interventions

Organisational and preventive interventions were shown to be effective in the Jones *et al.* study (Jones *et al.*, 1988) reported earlier, in terms of both staff stress levels and less litigation. Different ways of organising practice and training may also be effective: when house officers at the end of their two traditional 6-month rotations in different hospitals were compared to those in a new 12-month single-hospital rotation, only 10% of the latter group had above-threshold GHQ levels, compared to 25% of the traditional group (Firth-Cozens *et al.*, 2000). It is not surprising that staying in one organisation, reducing life events, and building up relationships and organisational knowledge are likely to create so much better mental health. The interventions are often easy and obvious – if the effects of stress on patient care are taken seriously, then much can be achieved.

The doctors themselves can have preventive stress management and support; for example, by:

- stress-management training
- alcohol and drug awareness from undergraduate days
- mentoring and career counselling
- having their own general practitioner
- by undergraduate and postgraduate training establishments recording student mental health problems (Brewin & Firth-Cozens, 1997) and behaviour (Papadakis *et al.*, 2004) as potential indicators of later problems and so dealing with them early.

A study of pre-registration house officers has concluded (Paice *et al.*, 2002) that interventions to reduce their stress would include better supervision in the first few weeks in post, more time to discuss issues with colleagues, and more personal time with friends and family.

Getting individual help

Doctors, like anyone else, need help when they are in difficulty. They should normally be advised to consult their general practitioner or be referred to an occupational health physician. Doctors frequently find it difficult to treat other doctors (*see* Chapter 1) and referral to more specialist agencies may be useful. There is a need for access to a raft of different forms of support and interventions such as a source of good assessment, self-help organisations, short- and long-term counselling, psychotherapy and psychiatry. Doctors have an ethical duty to take and follow advice if they know that their judgement or performance could be significantly affected by illness or its treatment. They should not rely on their own assessment of the risk to patients.

Rates of recovery

In terms of the ability of clinically depressed professionals to reduce symptoms significantly and maintain any changes made, recovery has shown to be reasonably long-term with brief psychotherapy (Firth & Shapiro, 1986). Doctors have been shown to recover quite well from alcohol abuse using Alcoholics Anonymous or its 12-step programme (Khantzian & Mack, 1994; Carlson & Dilts, 1994; Lloyd, 2002), and well-publicised access numbers for self-help organisations such as AA or Narcotics Anonymous may help to make this process more acceptable. Of 100 alcoholic doctors over a 21-year period, there was a 73% recovery rate over 17 years, primarily through abstinence and self-help group meetings (Lloyd, 2002). In studies of interventions with pilots who abuse alcohol, it is now thought possible to make informed predictions at an early date, after abstinence and recovery have begun, about the future continued success of an individual's rehabilitation, though frequent monitoring is maintained with this occupational group (Pakull, 2002).

Conclusions

Stress and depression are a cause for concern in health service staff, particularly doctors because of the effects on the doctor, on the organisation in terms of costs, and on the patient in terms of reduced quality of care. We have considerable evidence of the individual and organisational causes of these problems, and a number of evidence-based primary and secondary interventions to ameliorate them. Good human resource management will continue to address this task as a matter of priority.

References

Angres DH *et al*. (2003) Psychiatric comorbidity and physicians with substance use disorders: a comparison between the 1980s and 1990s. *Journal of Addictive Diseases*. **22**(3): 79–87.

Baldwin PJ, Dodd M and Wrate RW (1997) Young doctors' health – I How do working conditions affect attitudes, health and performance? *Social Science and Medicine*. **45**(1): 35–40.

Birch D, Ashton H and Kamali F (1998) Alcohol, drinking, illicit drug use, and stress in junior house officers in north-east England. *The Lancet*. **352**(9130): 785–6.

Bissell L and Skorina JK (1987) One hundred alcoholic women in medicine. *JAMA*. **257**(21): 2939–44.

Blatt SJ and Zuroff DC (1992) Interpersonal relatedness and self-definition: two proto-types for depression. *Clinical Psychology Review*. **12**(5): 527–62.

Boisaubin EV and Levine RE (2001) Identifying and assisting the impaired physician. *American Journal of the Medical Sciences*. **322**(1): 31–6.

Brewin C and Firth-Cozens J (1997) Dependency and self-criticism as predictors of depression in young doctors. *Journal of Occupational Health Psychology*. **2**(3): 242–6.

Broadbent DE *et al*. (1982) The Cognitive Failures Questionnaire (CFQ) and its correlates. *British Journal of Clinical Psychology*. **21**(1): 1–16.

Brooke D, Edwards G and Taylor C (1991) Addiction as an occupational hazard: 144 doctors with drug and alcohol problems. *British Journal of Addiction*. **86**(8): 1011–16.

Caplan RP (1994) Stress, anxiety and depression in hospital consultants, general practitioners, and senior health service managers. *BMJ*. **309**(6964): 1261–3.

Carlson HB and Dilts SL (1994) Physicians with substance abuse problems and their recovery environment: a survey. *Journal of Substance Abuse Treatment*. **11**: 113–19.

Carter AJ and West MA (1999) Sharing the burden: team work in health care setting. In: J Firth-Cozens and RL Payne (eds) *Stress in Health Professionals: psychological and organisational causes and interventions*. John Wiley & Sons, Chichester, pp. 191–202.

Carthey J *et al*. (2003) Behavioural markers of surgical excellence. *Safety Science*. **41**(5): 409–25.

Caspi A *et al*. (1997) Personality differences predict health-risk behaviors in young adulthood: evidence from a longitudinal study. *Journal of Personality and Social Psychology*. **73**(5): 1052–63.

Center C *et al*. (2003) Confronting depression and suicide in physicians: a consensus statement. *JAMA*. **289**(23): 3161–7.

Crow SM *et al*. (2003) A prescription for the rogue doctor: part I – begin with diagnosis. *Clinical Orthopaedics and Related Research*. **411**: 334–9.

Czander WM (1993) *The Psychodynamics of Work and Organizations: theory and application*. Guilford Press, New York.

Derogatis LR, Lipman RS and Covi L (1973) SCL-90: an outpatient psychiatric rating scale – preliminary report. *Psychopharmacology Bulletin*. **9**(1): 13–20.

DiMatteo MR *et al*. (1993) Physicians' characteristics influence patients' adherence to medical treatment: results from the medical outcomes study. *Health Psychology*. **12**(2): 93–102.

Domenighetti G *et al*. (1991) Psychoactive drug use among medical doctors is higher than in the general population. *Social Science and Medicine*. **33**(3): 269–74.

Dumelow C, Littlejohns P and Griffiths S (2000) Relation between a career and family life for English hospital consultants: qualitative, semistructured interview study. *BMJ*. **320**(7247): 1437–40.

Dunbar M, Ford G, Hunt K and Der G (2000) A confirmatory factor analysis of the Hospital Anxiety and Depression Scale: comparing empirically and theoretically derived structures. *British Journal of Clinical Psychology*. **39**: 79–94.

Farmer JF (2002) Return to work for junior doctors after ill-health. *Medical Journal of Australia*. **177**(1 Suppl): S27–S29.

Firth J and Shapiro D (1986) An evaluation of psychotherapy for job-related distress. *Journal of Occupational Psychology*. **59**: 221–33.

Firth-Cozens J (1992) The role of early family experiences in the perception of organizational stress: fusing clinical and organizational perspectives. *Journal of Occupational and Organizational Psychology*. **65**(1): 61–75.

Firth-Cozens J (1995) Sources of stress in junior doctors and general practitioners. *Yorkshire Medicine*. **7**: 10–13.

Firth-Cozens J (1997) Depression in doctors. In: C Katona and MM Robertson (eds) *Depression and Physical Illness*. John Wiley & Sons, Chichester, pp. 95–111.

Firth-Cozens J (1998) Individual and organizational predictors of depression in general practitioners. *British Journal of General Practice*. **48**(435): 1647–51.

Firth-Cozens J (1999a) *Training in the Pre-registration House Officer Year (Report 1)*. North Thames Department of Postgraduate Medicine and Dental Education, London.

Firth-Cozens J (1999b) The psychological problems of doctors. In: J Firth-Cozens and RL Payne (eds) *Stress in Health Professionals: psychological and organisational causes and interventions*. John Wiley & Sons, Chichester, pp. 79–91.

Firth-Cozens J et al. (2000) The effect of 1-year rotations on stress in preregistration house officers. *Hospital Medicine*. **61**(12): 859–60.

Firth-Cozens J (2001) Interventions to improve physicians' well-being and patient care. *Social Science and Medicine*. **52**(2): 215–22.

Firth-Cozens J (2004) New Research on Stress in Doctors. Paper given at La Fundación Galatea Conference, January 2004, Madrid.

Firth-Cozens J and Bonanno D (1999) *What is Training Like? Views on training and support for full-time and flexible specialist registrars*. Report to Postgraduate Deanery of Medicine, Newcastle.

Firth-Cozens J and Greenhalgh J (1997) Doctors' perceptions of the links between stress and lowered clinical care. *Social Science and Medicine*. **44**(7): 1017–22.

Firth-Cozens J and Morrison LA (1989) Sources of stress and ways of coping in junior house officers. *Stress Medicine*. **5**(2): 121–6.

Firth-Cozens J, Lema VC and Firth RA (1999) Speciality choice, stress and personality: their relationships over time. *Hospital Medicine*. **60**(10): 751–5.

Firth-Cozens J, Midgley S and Burges C (1999) Questionnaire survey of post-traumatic stress disorder in doctors involved in the Omagh bombing. *BMJ*. **319**(7225): 1609.

Flaherty JA and Richman JA (1993) Substance use and addiction among medical students, residents and physicians. *Psychiatric Clinics of North America*. **16**(1): 189–97.

Frank E et al. (2000) Correlates of physicians' prevention-related practices. Finding from the Women Physicians' Health Study. *Archives of Family Medicine*. **9**(4): 359–67.

Gerber LA (1983) *Married to their Careers: career and family dilemmas in doctors' lives*. Tavistock, New York.

Ghodse H (2000) Doctors and their health – who heals the healers? In: H Ghodse, S Mann and P Johnson (eds) *Doctors and their Health*. Reed Healthcare Limited, Sutton, pp. 10–14.

Goldberg DP (1978) *Manual of the General Health Questionnaire*. NFER, Windsor.

Harrison D and Chick J (1994) Trends in alcoholism among male doctors in Scotland. *Addiction*. **89**(12): 1613–17.

Hawton K et al. (2001) Suicide in doctors: a study of risk according to gender, seniority and specialty in medical practitioners in England and Wales 1979–95. *Journal of Epidemiology and Community Health*. **55**(5): 296–300.

Heather N and Kaner E (2003) Brief interventions against excessive alcohol consumption. In: DA Warrell, TM Cox and JD Firth (eds) *Oxford Textbook of Medicine* (4e, vol. 3). Oxford Medical Publications, Oxford.

Helmreich RL and Willhelm JA (1991) Outcomes of crew resource management training. *The International Journal of Aviation Psychology*. **1**(4): 287–300.

Hem E (2004) *Suicidal Behaviour in Some Human Service Occupations with Special Emphasis on Physicians and Police: a nationwide study* [online]. Unipub AS, Oslo. Available at: www.legeforeningen.no/?id=46822 [Accessed 6 October 2004].

Henquet C, Krabbendam L, Spauwen C, Lieb R et al. (2005) Prospective cohort study of cannabis use: predisposition for psychosis and psychotic symptoms in young people. *BMJ*. **330**(7481): 11.

Holahan CJ *et al.* (2004) Unipolar depression, life context vulnerabilities, and drinking to cope. *Journal of Consulting and Clinical Psychology.* **72**(2): 269–75.

Houston DM and Allt SK (1997) Psychological distress and error making among junior house officers. *British Journal of Health Psychology.* **12**(2): 141–51.

Jones JW *et al.* (1988) Stress and medical malpractice: organizational risk assessment and intervention. *Journal of Applied Psychology.* **73**(4): 727–35.

Kapur N, Borrill C and Stride C (1998) Psychological morbidity and job satisfaction in hospital consultants and junior house officers: multicentre, cross sectional survey. *BMJ.* **317**(7157): 511–12.

Khantzian EJ and Mack JE (1994) How AA works and why it's important for clinicians to understand. *Journal of Substance Abuse Treatment.* **11**: 77–92.

Koeske GF, Kirk SA and Koeske RD (1993) Coping with job stress: Which strategies work best? *Journal of Occupational and Organizational Psychology.* **66**(4): 319–35.

Kohut H (1971) *The Analysis of the Self: a systematic approach to the psychoanalytic treatment of narcissistic personality disorders.* International Universities Press, New York.

Lindeman S *et al.* (1999) Treatment of mental disorders in seven physicians committing suicide. *Crisis.* **20**(2): 86–9.

Linn LS *et al.* (1995) Physician and patient satisfaction as factors related to the organization of internal medicine group practices. *Medical Care.* **23**(10): 1171–8.

Lloyd G (2002) One hundred alcoholic doctors: a 21 year follow-up. *Alcohol and Alcoholism.* **37**(4): 370–4.

Michelsen H and Bildt C (2003) Psychosocial conditions on and off the job and psychological ill health: depressive symptoms, impaired psychological wellbeing, heavy consumption of alcohol. *Occupational and Environmental Medicine.* **60**(7): 489–96.

Newton J *et al.* (2004) Job dissatisfaction and early retirement: a qualitative study of general practitioners in the Northern Deanery. *Primary Health Care Research and Development.* **5**(1): 68–76.

North FM *et al.* (1996) Psychosocial work environment and sickness absence among British civil servants: the Whitehall II study. *American Journal of Public Health.* **86**: 332–40.

Paice E, Rutter H, Wetherell M, Winder B and McManus IC (2002) Stressful incidents, stress and coping strategies in the pre-registration house officer year. *Medical Education.* **36**: 56–65.

Pakull B (2002) The federal aviation administration's role in evaluation of pilots and others with alcoholism or drug addiction. *Occupational Medicine.* **17**(2): 221–6, iv.

Papadakis MA, Hodgson CS, Teherani A and Kohatsu ND (2004) Unprofessional behavior in medical school is associated with subsequent disciplinary action by a State Medical Board. *Academic Medicine.* **29**: 244–9.

Pattani S, Constantinovici N and Williams S (2001) Who retires early from the NHS because of ill health and what does it cost? A national cross sectional study. *BMJ.* **322**(7280): 208–9.

Payne R and Firth-Cozens J (1987) Introduction. In: R Payne and J Firth-Cozens (eds) *Stress in Health Professionals.* John Wiley & Sons, Chichester, pp. xv–xxiv.

Pirkis J and Burgess P (1998) Suicide and recency of health care contacts: a systematic review. *British Journal of Psychiatry.* **173**: 462–74.

Reason J (1988) Stress and cognitive failure. In: S. Fisher and J Reason (eds) *Handbook of Life Stress, Cognition and Health.* John Wiley & Sons, Chichester, pp. 405–21.

Richman JA (1992) Occupational stress, psychological vulnerability and alcohol-related problems over time in future physicians. *Alcoholism, Clinical and Experimental Research.* **16**(2): 166–71.

Roberts K (1990) Managing high reliability organizations. *California Management Review.* **32**(4):100–13.

Saunders JB *et al.* (1993) Development of the Alcohol Use Disorders Identification Test (AUDIT): WHO Collaborative Project on the early detection of persons with harmful alcohol consumption – II. *Addiction.* **88**(6): 791–804.

Sclare B (1979) Alcoholism in doctors. *British Journal of Alcohol & Alcoholism.* **14**: 181–96.

Simon GE and VonKorff M (1995) Recognition, management and outcomes of depression in primary care. *Archives of Family Medicine.* **4**(2): 99–105.

Strang J (1998) Missed problems and missed opportunities for addicted doctors. *BMJ.* **316**(7129): 405–6.

Tattersall AJ, Bennet P and Pugh S (1999) Stress and coping in hospital doctors. *Stress Medicine.* **15**(2): 109–13.

Thomas CB and Duszynski KR (1974) Closeness to parents and the family constellation in a prospective study of five disease states: suicide, mental illness, malignant tumour, hypertension and coronary heart disease. *Johns Hopkins Medical Journal.* **134**(5): 251–70.

Turner RJ and Lloyd DA (2004) Stress burden and the lifetime incidence of psychiatric disorder in young adults: racial and ethnic contrasts. *Archives of General Psychiatry.* **61**(5): 481–8.

Tyssen R *et al.* (2004) The process of suicidal planning among medical doctors: predictors in a longitudinal Norwegian sample. *Journal of Affective Disorders.* **80**(2–3): 191–8.

Vaillant GE, Sobowale NC and McArthur C (1972) Some psychological vulnerabilities of physicians. *New England Journal of Medicine.* **287**(8): 372–5.

Van Kleef GA, De Dreu CK and Manstead AS (2004) The interpersonal effects of anger and happiness in negotiations. *Journal of Personality and Social Psychology.* **86**(1): 57–76.

Vincent C (1996) Editorial: Needs of staff after serious incidents and during litigation. *Clinical Risk.* **2**: 179–80.

Wall TD *et al.* (1997) Minor psychiatric disorder in NHS trust staff: occupational and gender differences. *British Journal of Psychiatry.* **171**: 519–23.

Weinberg A and Creed F (2000) Stress and psychiatric disorder in healthcare professionals and hospital staff. *The Lancet.* **355**(9203): 533–7.

Weinger MB and Ancoli-Israel S (2002) Sleep deprivation and clinical performance. *JAMA.* **287**(8): 955–7.

Chapter 3

Misuse of drugs and alcohol

Hamid Ghodse and Susanna Galea

Introduction

Substance misuse problems are amongst the most prevalent of health factors affecting doctors' performance. For example, a survey of house officers revealed that 56% drank alcohol in excess of recommended safe weekly limits and 10% used illegal drugs (Brooks, 1998). Misuse of substances can affect a doctor's performance both directly and indirectly. Direct effects are largely dependent upon the type of substance misused and the nature and extent of misuse. Indirect effects include psychosocial complications such as financial difficulties, social withdrawal and isolation, involvement in criminal activity, and the blurring of professional boundaries.

Impairment in performance due to misuse of substances is difficult to detect, especially if substance use has not reached a level of dependency (i.e. use is frequent but not a daily occurrence).

The extent of the problem

The misuse of drugs and alcohol by doctors has been described in several studies. Stuart and Price (Stuart & Price, 2000) described the difficulties in investigating the epidemiological literature on such high risk groups. One of the main difficulties is related to variations in definitions used. Methodological difficulties include retrospective self-reporting, varying demographic characteristics of the sample, non-representativeness of respondents and under-reporting by respondents. Despite such difficulties it is clear that doctors and healthcare professionals are a recognised high risk group for substance misuse and its consequences (Bissell & Hagerman, 1984).

Studies comparing substance misuse among doctors with the general population frequently report higher prevalence rates among doctors. An early study reported that physicians were 30 to 100 times more likely than the general population to become addicted to narcotics (Brewster, 1986). Another study (Hughes *et al.*, 1992) reported that physicians in the US were more likely to use alcohol and prescription drugs, such as benzodiazepines, but less likely to use tobacco and illicit substances, such as cocaine and heroin, than the general population. The General Household Survey for Great Britain (Rickards *et al.*, 2004) did not give specific data on doctors but reported on drinking and smoking patterns in various socioeconomic levels, as defined by the *National Statistics Socio-Economic Classification* (Walker *et al.*, 2003). Those in managerial and professional occupations consumed 12.7 units of alcohol per week, compared to 11.3 for those in routine and manual occupations. Similarly, compared with those earning £200 or less per week, those with a weekly income of £1000 or more were twice as likely to have drunk more than 8 units for men and more than 6 units for women on at least one day in the previous week. Conversely, studies on the prevalence of tobacco smoking revealed that manual workers smoked more (33%) than professional workers (14%).

Studies comparing doctors to other professional people of a comparable educational status also identified doctors as a higher risk group. A prospective study (Vaillant *et al.*, 1970) of college graduates showed that those graduating in medicine subsequently used more psychoactive drugs than other graduates. However, there were no differences between graduates in relation to alcohol and cigarettes. The British Medical Association estimated that in the UK one in fifteen doctors suffered from drug or alcohol dependency (British Medical Association, 1988). US data show that 10–15% of physicians are likely to develop dependence in their lifetime (Hughes *et al.*, 1992; Bennett & O'Donovan, 2001).

A study (McGovern, Angre & Leon, 2000) comparing doctors in different specialities rated family practitioners as the group with highest prevalence (28.8%) of substance misuse. Then came internists (12%), psychiatrists, gynaecologists and physicians in emergency medicine. Another study (Hughes *et al.*, 1992) reported highest rates for psychiatrists (14.3%) and physicians in emergency medicine (12.4%), with the lowest rates among surgeons (5.5%).

In contrast to the studies mentioned earlier, there are reports of a higher prevalence of substance misuse among anaesthetists. At least one anaesthetist per month, over a 10-year period, presented with significant alcohol or drug misuse in the UK and Ireland (Berry *et al.*, 2000). It was suggested that anaesthetists have been over-represented in the literature (Winstock & Strang, 1999), or that overall the speciality made significant efforts to decrease substance misuse (Hughes *et al.*, 1992; Bennett & O'Donovan, 2001) or that identification encouraged anaesthetists eventually to change speciality (Hughes *et al.*, 1992; Bennett & O'Donovan, 2001).

The misused substance also varied among specialities (Hughes *et al.*, 1992). Misuse of opioids was more common amongst emergency medicine physicians, anaesthetists and pain specialists. On the other hand, benzodiazepine misuse was common among psychiatrists (26.3%) and marihuana use was more common among emergency medicine physicians (10.5%). Another study (Paris & Canavan, 1999) reported fentanyl as the substance of choice for anaesthetists.

Brook and others (1993) found differences in prevalence rates between consultant and non-consultant grades. The use of cocaine, cannabis and benzodiazepines was more prevalent among non-consultant grades (35%) than among consultants (4%). On the other hand, alcohol dependency was more common among consultants (63%) than non-consultants (30%).

Such epidemiological data give an indication of the extent and nature of substance misuse among doctors.

Why does the problem arise?

Several factors specific to doctors have been mentioned in the literature as possible aetiological factors for drug and alcohol misuse among doctors.

Stress, anxiety and burnout

Work-related stress, anxiety and burnout are thought to be factors significantly contributing to the misuse of substances with consequent impairment in work performance. Stress levels among doctors and other healthcare workers are higher than stress levels within the general population (Wall *et al.*, 1997), with about 30% of doctors at any point in time suffering from stress (Firth-Cozens, 1995; Paice, 2000).

Stress among doctors is not restricted to specific specialities or career levels, although some groups are considered to be more vulnerable than others. For instance, doctors within their first year of practice (Paice, 2000) and female doctors (Graske, 2003) tend to exhibit higher levels of psychological morbidity. Suicide rates are highest are among anaesthetists, general practitioners and psychiatrists (Graske, 2003).

Although the experience of stress is correlated with individual responses to difficult situations, the high standards and demands of the doctor's role potentiate the development of stress (Fox, Dwyer & Ganster, 1993). From medical student years, the doctor is encouraged and trained to perform a multitude of tasks at high standards. Admission of tiredness or difficulty in coping can be perceived as failure. Hence doctors are discouraged from disclosing problems, which can lead to isolation. Long hours of work, intensity of work and decreased hours of sleep are other intrinsic factors of the doctors' role which contribute to stress levels (*see* Chapter 8).

Other factors perceived by doctors as being responsible for stress are: difficulties in maintaining a balance between career demands and personal life; fear of making mistakes; fear of litigation; difficulties in relationships between the hierarchical career levels; and dealing with patients in general (Firth-Cozens, 1995).

Stress levels among doctors are also dependent upon organisational factors. For instance, large organisations tend to be associated with higher proportions of stress than smaller health organisations (Aiken, Sloane & Sochalski, 1998; Firth-Cozens, 2000), and teaching hospitals rather than non-teaching hospitals (Paice, 2000).

Burnout has also been frequently described in the literature as correlating with stress and drug or alcohol use among doctors. Burnout is defined as 'a syndrome of emotional exhaustion involving the development of a negative self concept, negative job attitudes and loss of concern and feeling for clients' (Pines & Maslach, 1978). It is 'a state of physical, emotional and mental exhaustion, caused by long-term involvement in situations that are emotionally demanding' (Pines & Aronson, 1988; Roberts, 2000). Rates ranging from 25% to 76% have been reported (Shanafelt *et al.*, 2002; Ramirez *et al.*, 1995; Lemkau, Rafferty & Gordon, 1994; Grassi & Magnani, 2000) among doctors. Post-traumatic stress disorder has also been given particular attention, with doctors considered to be a vulnerable group (Persaud, 2005).

Stress, anxiety and burnout play an aetiological role in substance misuse and decreased performance in doctors. Firth-Cozens (Firth-Cozens, 1995; Firth-Cozens, 2000) found that 65% of senior doctors used alcohol as a coping strategy, with 11% using it 'frequently' for this purpose. Excessive drinking and use of mood-altering drugs has also been reported as being associated with burnout (Cathebras *et al.*, 2004; Roberts, 2000) and post-traumatic stress disorder (Persaud, 2005).

Easy access and self-prescribing

Self-prescribing is common among doctors, especially with general practitioners. Doctors frequently carry out self-diagnosis and unsupervised self-treatment contributing to substance misuse and dependency. Several studies reported that the extent of self-prescribing among doctors was cause for concern (Hughes *et al.*, 1992; Toyry *et al.*, 2000; Forsythe, Calnan & Wall, 1999). Another study (Vaillant, Brighton & McArthur, 1970) reported that self-medication with prescription drugs, mainly sedatives, amphetamines and tranquillizers, was responsible for a third of the time spent by doctors as patients in hospital. Joranson *et al.* (2000) found that 42.1% of male doctors and 52.9% of female doctors had written self-prescriptions within the past year. Self-prescribing and access to drugs from other sources contribute to easy access to substances.

Attributes of the doctor

Choosing one's profession depends partly on personal attributes. Early childhood experiences are thought to contribute to the choice of becoming a healthcare professional. Emotional neglect in childhood is believed to contribute to the choice of working in the care field (Brooke, 2000). Evidence (Vaillant, Brighton & McArthur, 1970; Firth-Cozens, 1992) suggests that traumatic childhood experiences, such as parental divorce and maternal death, are associated with higher stress levels and increased misuse of substances.

Some personality traits are also thought to contribute to increased psychological morbidity. Doctors' work culture promotes perfectionism and self-criticism, which in turn are predictors of stress and depression (Firth-Cozens, 1998). Idealism, high levels of self-discipline, rigidity in behaviour and high levels of empathy all contribute to difficulty in coping (Graske, 2003).

Denial and avoidance are common strategies adopted by doctors. This is reflected in delays in seeking help as well as continuing to work despite ill health (Graske, 2003). A quote from a recent article highlights the issue: 'often doctors will recognise their own symptoms but tend to delay seeking help because of factors such as denial, fear of stigma and a difficulty seeing him or herself as a patient' (Brettingham, 2005). Avoidance strategies contribute to stress and ill health (Firth-Cozens, 2000; Firth-Cozens & Morrison, 1989). The work culture of 'stoicism, detachment and denial of our own vulnerabilities' (Graske, 2003) sets off a vicious circle of stigma, isolation, secrecy and under-detection.

Evidence on the contribution of knowledge of the effects of mind-altering substances to under-detection is sparse.

Social attributes

Factors associated with increased substance misuse within society will also affect doctors. Globally, the misuse of drugs is on the increase, with global attitudinal and cultural changes (United Nations Office for Drug Control and Crime Prevention, 2000). Studies revealing high prevalence rates of substance misuse (Brooks, 1998) reflect such global increases. However, there is little evidence showing increases in prevalence among doctors over time. Other factors, such as weekly income, have also been associated with substance misuse. The General Household Survey (Rickards *et al.*, 2004) identified that those with a higher weekly income drank more. Doctors are generally higher earners, making them more susceptible.

Although contributory factors are subjective, awareness of common contributors facilitates early detection and prevention. Nevertheless each doctor needs to be assessed individually.

Effects of drugs and alcohol on performance

Poor performance related to drug and alcohol misuse is the result of both the direct effects of the substance itself and the indirect effects such as associated financial difficulties, relationship problems and criminal activity. The same factors that cause misuse of drugs and alcohol in doctors can also have significant impact on their professional performance.

Direct substance effects

Substances exert their effects through complex biological pathways. Different substances have different chemical and pharmacological properties which affect different parts of the central nervous system. Furthermore, drugs and alcohol have rewarding and reinforcing properties which give them their addictive potential.

Sedative and hypnotic substances such as alcohol, opiates and benzodiazepines may directly influence a doctor's performance through their depressant effects. Alertness and co-ordination are affected to varying degrees depending upon the nature and extent of substance misuse. Similar dangerous direct effects such as increased activity and impaired attention can be observed with use of stimulants, such as amphetamines and cocaine.

Doctor-centred factors

The aetiological factors mentioned in the previous section, such as stress levels, burnout, psychological traits and experiences, all contribute to both substance misuse and impaired performance. Substance use also potentiates further stress and ill health. The resultant impact is gradual deterioration in performance.

Compared to other doctors, those experiencing burnout are significantly more likely to engage in suboptimal patient care (32% compared to 11%) (Shanafelt *et al.*, 2002). The evidence indicates a link between stress, substance misuse, job dissatisfaction and underperformance (Firth-Cozens, 2000; Jones *et al.*, 1988; DeMatteo *et al.*, 1993) (*see* Chapters 2 and 5).

Work-centred factors

High standards and demands, combined with a culture of denial and avoidance, provide fertile ground for substance misuse, underperformance and suboptimal patient care, particularly if this is associated with denial. Inadequate support and training are associated with feelings of inadequacy, stress and misuse of substances (Chrome, 1999). Self-diagnosis and self-prescribing, although perhaps resulting in fewer sickness days, are themselves performance issues. General Medical Council guidance is that doctors should not treat themselves or their families (General Medical Council, 1998). Many organisations have their own policies which prohibit such practices, which may trigger capability procedures at work.

Non-work factors

Misuse of drugs and alcohol is associated with several complications. For instance, relationship problems, self-neglect, financial problems and engagement in criminal behaviours in the process of obtaining substances can also contribute to poor performance at work. Difficulties with colleagues due to inappropriate behaviour and an attempt at secrecy may also lead to isolation and impaired performance. Furthermore, traumatic life events may have been the trigger for a doctor's misuse of substances. Hence underperformance may have wide implications.

Prevention and early detection

Preventative measures at both organisational and individual levels also facilitate early detection of drug and or alcohol misuse by doctors.

Training plays an important role in prevention and early detection. Education for healthcare professionals increases awareness of the problem, such that substance use is thought of and talked about, rather than being stigmatised and masked. Healthcare professionals need to be aware of the risks associated with use of substances by a doctor. They need to be aware of the possible aetiological factors which serve to initiate and maintain substance misuse. They need to know what to do if they suspect or are aware that a colleague is misusing substances. SCODA, a charity for drug abuse, reported that most medical schools in the UK provided limited formal training on addictive behaviour, with the national average being only 7 hours (half the average time reported in 1987) (SCODA, 1999). More time should be spent in heightening awareness in medical students and doctors for their own benefit as well as their patients'.

Firth-Cozens (Firth-Cozens, 2000) provides a systems model looking at appropriate intervention at various levels; she recognises the role of mentoring, supervision and counselling. Alcohol and substance misuse can more easily be prevented and detected by giving consideration to high-risk factors. The importance of appropriate support was highlighted in a survey of pre-registration house officers (Paice, 2000). Issues such as high levels of self-criticism and mood difficulties can be addressed and counselling on career changes may be considered appropriate. Recognition of ineffective coping strategies is also of utmost importance.

At an organisational level, the regular monitoring of key performance indicators (Cornelius & Gooch, 2001), such as record keeping, application of evidence-based approaches, adherence to standards, patient satisfaction reports, complaints by other healthcare professionals, etc., facilitate early detection of difficulties, as do risk management procedures and incident reporting.

They may not, however, necessarily identify that the underlying problem is the misuse of substances. A non-judgemental management style with incident monitoring is likely to facilitate communication and early detection. A 'no-blame' and nurturing culture supports a safe communicative environment.

An alternative approach is the routine and/or random screening for drug and alcohol misuse. Within the US the practice is mandatory; however, this is not the case in the UK. The effectiveness of such screening procedures is questionable and would need to be accompanied by appropriate supportive structures. Mandatory screening can be perceived as punitive with potential legal implications, further enhancing masking, denial and isolation. However, if mandatory screening was linked with supportive schemes, the perception might be different. The question of identifying an effective approach relies upon weighing risks against benefits at local and national levels. A statement by the deputy chairman of the British Medical Association's Junior Doctors Committee highlights the main issues: 'if there was evidence that some sort of screening of NHS staff produced the best outcome, then it should be considered' (Brooks, 1998). It is clear that increased vigilance is needed, but the process of vigilance may need to be selected according to local needs.

Intervention

Effective clinical and managerial management is necessary at individual and organisational levels.

The success of interventions is dependent upon the motivational level of the individual. Self-prescribing, easy access, stigma and isolation, etc. facilitate doctors remaining in the 'pre-contemplative' and 'contemplative' stages of change (Prochaska & DiClemente, 1982) for longer than others. 'Pre-contemplation' is not just that the doctor does not reflect on the problem, but that neither do employers, health authorities or society as a whole. Society does not wish to accept that its doctors may suffer impairment or to feel let down by its authority figures; fellow doctors also do not wish to accept such impairment. Hence, doctors are continuously encouraged to remain within the pre-contemplative and contemplative stages of change for relatively long periods of time.

Special services specifically targeting addicted doctors are an important requirement within various societies (Bennett & O'Donovan, 2001; Strang *et al.*, 1998). Treating doctors within mainstream services does not facilitate engagement and compliance. Doctors may find it difficult to change role from 'doctor' to 'patient' and being treated within mainstream services makes this role-shift more difficult to adjust to.

Doctors need to be aware of and have easy access to existing services. Information on organisations providing a service to doctors needs to be readily available for all healthcare professionals. Examples of such organisations include: the Sick Doctors' Trust, National Counselling for Sick Doctors and International Doctors in Alcoholics Anonymous. Detoxification and rehabilitation programmes need to be highly specialised to cater for doctors' needs. Paris and Canavan (Paris & Canavan, 1999) reported on relapse rates of around 40% following detoxification and rehabilitation, whereas the Sick Doctors' Trust reported relapse rates of only 4.4% at five-year follow-ups (Joiner, 2000).

The 'doctor–doctor' relationship

Effective assessment and treatment depends upon the 'doctor–doctor' relationship. The reliability of the substance misuse history taken by the professional is dependent on whether the 'doctor–doctor' relationship nurtures trust, safety and respect of autonomy. Concerns of the addicted doctor about record keeping and breaches in confidentiality potentially encourage further masking and denial. The treating physician needs to be highly skilled to perform the doctor's role and advise accordingly, whilst respecting the knowledge, psychological struggle and role difficulties of the ill doctor.

Research

Research on misuse of drugs and alcohol by doctors is relatively sparse. Doctors are a vulnerable group for several reasons but the roles played by the misuse of both drugs and alcohol are still unclear. The relative risk of aetiological factors and the dynamic interplay of such factors need further clarification. Knowledge of relapse indicators or determinants of relapse, both long-term and short-term, will assist in the development of effective services. The impact of education and increased awareness of doctors' vulnerabilities to the misuse of substances can also inform further specialised programmes.

Conclusion

The impact of drug and/or alcohol misuse on a doctor's performance has been discussed in this chapter. Prevalence studies indicate that the problem is common, with potential significant and harmful consequences to society. The culture of a doctor's world, as well as intrinsic factors within the professional, make doctors a vulnerable cohort for substance use. Factors such as self-prescribing and easy access potentiate the problem. Others such as stigma, denial and self-criticism impede early detection. Specialised services for addicted doctors are the way forward. However, further research is required to inform the process and implementation of such services.

References

Aiken LH, Sloane DM and Sochalski J (1998) Hospital organisation and outcomes. *Quality in Health Care*. 7: 222–6.

Bennett J and O'Donovan D (2001) Substance misuse by doctors, nurses and other healthcare workers. *Current Opinion in Psychiatry*. 14: 195–9.

Berry CB, Crome IB, Plant M and Plant M (2000) Substance misuse amongst anaesthetists in the United Kingdom and Ireland – the results of a study commissioned by the Association of Anaesthetists of Great Britain & Ireland. *Anaesthesia*. 55: 946–52.

Bissell L and Hagerman P (1984) *Alcoholism in the Professions*. Oxford University Press, New York.

Brettingham M (2005) DIY Medicine. *BMA News*. **January** 1: 6.

Brewster JM (1986) Prevalence of alcohol and other drug problems among physicians. *Journal of the American Medical Association*. **255**: 1913–20.

British Medical Association (1988) *The Misuse of Alcohol and Other Drugs by Doctors*. Working Group on Misuse of Alcohol and other Drugs by Doctors, British Medical Association, London.

Brook D, Edwards G and Andrews T (1993) Doctors and substance misuse: types of doctors, types of problems. *Addiction*. **88**(5): 655–63.

Brooke D (2000) Doctors and their health – drug and alcohol problems. In: H Ghodse, S Mann and P Johnson (eds) *Doctors and their Health*. Reed Healthcare Limited, Surrey, pp. 30–5.

Brooks A (1998) Many junior doctors misuse drugs and drink excessively. *BMJ*. **317**(7160): 700.

Cathebras P, Begon A, Laporte S, Bois C and Truchot D (2004) Burnout among French general practitioners. *Presse Med*. **33**(22): 1569–74.

Chrome I (1999) The trouble with training: Substance misuse education in British medical schools revisited: what are the issues? *Education Prevention and Policy*. 6: 111–25.

Cornelius N and Gooch L (2001) Performance management: strategy, systems and rewards. In: N Cornelius (ed.) *Human Resource Management: a managerial perspective* (2e). Thomson Learning, London, pp. 141–78.

DeMatteo MR, Sherbourne CD, Hays RD and Ordway L (1993) Physicians' characteristics influence patients' adherence to medical treatment: results from the medical outcomes study. *Health Psychology*. **12**: 93–102.

Firth-Cozens J (2000) Interventions to improve physicians' well-being and patient care. *Social Science and Medicine*. **52**(2001): 215–22.

Firth-Cozens J (1998) Individual and organisational predictors of depression in general practitioners. *British Journal of General Practice*. **48**: 1647–51.

Firth-Cozens J (1995) Sources of stress in junior doctors and general practitioners. *Yorkshire Medicine*. **7**: 10–13.

Firth-Cozens J (1992) The role of early family experience in the perception of organisation stress: fusing clinical and organisation perspectives. *Journal of Occupational and Organisational Psychology*. **65**: 61–75.

Firth-Cozens J and Morrison L (1989) Sources of stress and ways of coping in junior house officers. *Stress Medicine*. **5**: 121–6.

Forsythe M, Calnan M and Wall B (1999) Doctors as patients: postal survey examining consultants' and general practitioners' adherence to guidelines. *BMJ*. **319**(7210): 605–8.

Fox ML, Dwyer DJ and Ganster DC (1993) Effects of stressful job demands and control on physiological and attitudinal outcomes in a hospital setting. *Academy of Management Journal*. **36**(2): 289–318.

General Medical Council (1998) Doctors should not treat themselves or their families. Available at: www.gmc-uk.org/standards/default.htm.

Graske J (2003) Improving the mental health of doctors. *BMJ Careers*. **13 December**: s188.

Grassi L and Magnani K (2000) Psychiatric morbidity and burnout in the medical profession: an Italian study of general practitioners and hospital physicians. *Psychother Psychosom*. **69**: 329–34.

Hughes PH, Brandenburg N, Baldwin DC Jr, Storr CL, Williams KM, Anthony JC and Sheehan DV (1992) Prevalence of substance use among US physicians. *Journal of the American Medical Association*. **267**(17): 2333–9.

Joiner I (2000) The Sick Doctors Trust – Addicted Physicians Physicians Programme. In: H Ghodse, S Mann and P Johnson (eds) *Doctors and their Health*. Reed Healthcare Limited, Surrey, pp. 87–95.

Jones JW, Barge BN, Steffy BD, Fay LM, Kunz LK and Wuebker LJ (1988) Stress and medical malpractice: organizational risk assessment and intervention. *Journal of Applied Psychology*. **4**: 727–35.

Joranson D, Ryan K, Gilson A and Dahl J (2000) Trends in medical use and abuse of opioid analgesics. *Journal of the American Medical Association*. **283**: 1710–14.

Lemkau J, Rafferty J and Gordon R Jr (1994) Burnout and career-choice regret among family practice physicians in early practice. *Family Practitioners Res Journal*. **14**: 213–22.

McGovern M, Angre D and Leon S (2000) Characteristics of physicians presenting for assessment at a behavioural health centre. *Journal of Addictive Disorders*. **19**: 59–73.

Paice E (2000) Early identification, diagnosis and response. In: H Ghodse, S Mann and P Johnson (eds) *Doctors and their Health*. Reed Healthcare Limited, Surrey, pp. 21–9.

Paris R and Canavan D (1999) Physician substance abuse impairment: anesthesiologists vs other specialities. *Journal of Addictive Disorders*. **18**: 1–7.

Persaud R (2005) Post-traumatic stress disorder in doctors. *BMJ Careers*. **26 February**: 86–7.

Pines A and Aronson E (1988) *Career Burnout: causes and cures*. Free Press, New York.

Pines A and Maslach C (1978) Characteristics of staff burnout in mental health settings. *Hospital & Community Psychiatry*. **29**: 233–7.

Prochaska JO and DiClemente CC (1982) Transtheoretical therapy: toward a more integrative model of change. *Psychotherapy: theory, research and practice*. **19**: 276–88.

Ramirez AJ, Graham J, Richards MA, Cull A, Gregory WM, Leaning MS *et al.* (1995) Burnout and psychiatric disorder among cancer clinicians. *British Journal of Cancer.* 71: 1263–9.

Rickards L, Fox K, Roberts C, Fletcher L and Goddard E (2004) *Living in Britain, No. 31: results from the 2002 General Household Survey.* Office of National Statistics, The Stationery Office, HMSO, London.

Roberts G (2000) Burnout and how to survive it. In: H Ghodse, S Mann and P Johnson (eds) *Doctors and their Health.* Reed Healthcare Limited, Surrey, pp. 36–43.

SCODA (1999) *Drug Training Call for Trainee Doctors.* Reported in BBC News, 15 December 1999.

Shanafelt TD, Bradley KA, Wipf JE and Back AL (2002) Burnout and self-reported patient care in an internal residency program. *Annals of Internal Medicine.* 136(5): 358–67.

Strang J, Wilks M, Wells B and Marshall J (1998) Missed problems and missed opportunities for addicted doctors. *BMJ.* 316: 405–6.

Stuart GL and Price LH (2000) Recent developments in populations at risk for substance abuse. *Current Opinion in Psychiatry.* 13: 315–20.

Toyry S, Rasanen K, Kujala S *et al.* (2000) Self-reported health, illness, and self-care among Finnish physicians: a national survey. *Archives of Family Medicine.* 9: 1079–85.

United Nations Office for Drug Control and Crime Prevention (2000) *World Drug Report 2000.* Oxford University Press, Oxford.

Vaillant G, Brighton J and McArthur C (1970) Physicians' use of mood-altering drugs: a 20-year follow-up report. *New England Journal of Medicine.* 282: 365–70.

Walker *et al.* (2003) *Living in Britain: results from the 2001 General Household Survey: Appendix E.* Office of National Statistics, The Stationery Office, HMSO, London.

Wall TD, Bolden RI, Borrill CS, West M, Carter AJ, Golya DA, Hardy GE, Haynes CE, Rick JE and Shapiro D (1997) Minor psychiatric disorders in NHS trust staff: occupational and gender differences. *British Journal of Psychiatry.* 171: 519–23.

Winstock A and Strang J (1999) Alternative ways of using and abusing drugs and the complicity of doctors. *Hospital Medicine.* 60: 165–8.

Chapter 4

Cognitive impairment and performance

Kirstie Gibson, Luke Kartsounis and Michael Kopelman

Key cognitive skills required in medical practice

The General Medical Council clearly states the important competencies for doctors in its core publication *Good Medical Practice* (General Medical Council, 2001).

The areas of competency include:

1 Conducting a consultation, taking a history and performing an examination to determine a diagnosis.
2 Deciding on appropriate treatment options, arranging further investigations to confirm or refute a diagnosis.
3 Recognising a medical emergency and taking action.
4 Knowing the limits of knowledge and when to make a referral.

The above four competencies require motivation to do a proficient job, memory, attention, concentration and abilities to plan, organise and monitor behaviour, collectively referred to as 'executive skills'. The competent doctor needs to have a sound and up-to-date knowledge base of their areas of practice and specialty, as well as psychological attributes that support normal human interactions. Specifically, the following capabilities are conducive to good practice:

Table 4.1 Capabilities conducive to good practice

Required skill/competency	Required cognitive function
Keeping clear records	Requires memory and the ability to write understandable English that is legible
Being able to communicate with patients, relatives and other colleagues	Ability to understand incoming words and concepts and the ability to formulate a response and speak coherently Requires normal social behaviour
Detect and manage patient distress Behave in a polite, considerate and truthful manner	Requires empathy, emotional control and the ability to consider others' feelings
Safe prescribing of medicines	Requires memory, decision making and ability to write a prescription clearly and calculate medication doses
Keeping up to date with new developments and carrying out audit and review	Requires 'executive skills' of motivation, prioritising and learning new material
Must not demonstrate any improper sexual or aggressive behaviour	Requires normal social behaviour
Being able to give clear advice in areas of diagnosis, treatment and prognosis	Requires clear thought, speech and ability to answer questions.

5 Keeping clear patient records needs memory and the ability to write understandable English that is legible.
6 Being able to communicate with patients, relatives and other colleagues needs
understanding of incoming words and concepts and the ability to formulate a
response and speak coherently. It also requires normal social behaviour.
7 Detecting and managing patient distress needs empathy and the ability to
consider others' feelings.
8 Being able to safely prescribe medication involves memory and decision making
plus the ability to write a prescription clearly and calculate doses.
9 Keeping up to date and taking part in audit requires executive skills of motivation, prioritising and learning new material.
10 Behaving in a polite, considerate and truthful way calls for emotional control.
11 Not demonstrating any improper sexual or aggressive behaviour requires normal social functioning.
12 Being able to give clear advice in areas of diagnosis, treatment and prognosis
necessitates clear thought, speech and ability to answer questions.

As in most other jobs, the integrity of cognitive skills is central to competency in
medical occupations. In their qualification exams, medical students are assessed
for memory (facts and their application plus pattern recognition), problem-solving
abilities, stamina (length of course and amount of material to know) and competency in practical areas of history taking and examination. Until recently, once
doctors had qualified and passed their relevant postgraduate exams, they might not
be formally assessed by a third party again in their careers. This is in contrast to
commercial pilots who have to undergo an annual proficiency test and 6-month
medical if aged over 40 years to receive a licence renewal (Joint Aviation Authority,
2004). But medicine is catching up, with the introduction of systems of professional
appraisal, audit and clinical governance which are aimed at reducing this gap in
performance assessment, which in some cases may identify underperformance that
may give cause for concern.

However, the public is more likely to complain than in the past if individuals feel
the doctor is not listening or is incompetent and the exploration of a complaint may
also identify performance problems. The GMC also makes it clear that it is a doctor's
duty to report a colleague who they feel is not performing in a professional way. As a
result cognitive deficiencies may first come to light via the GMC or NHS management system. A paper by Turnbull *et al.* (2000) used a neuropsychological screening
battery to assess cognitive impairment in 27 physicians being assessed for competency to practise. About a third of physicians who performed poorly on the
competency assessment were also found to have neuropsychological impairment
on testing. This work raised the issue of whether a neuropsychological screening
procedure for underperforming doctors should be developed, although there is no
standard battery of tests available for any particular condition. The current approach to assessment is explained in the section on 'Neuropsychological and
neuropsychiatric assessments' in this chapter.

Memory is a key ability involving both episodic (day-to-day) and semantic
(knowledge-based) aspects. Much of medical training is based on the acquisition
and application of new knowledge, and so a large knowledge base is progressively
acquired from the first days in medical school onwards. The process of diagnosis
involves being able to remember physical signs and symptoms and draw up a list of

possible diagnoses. By a process of logic, experience and assessment of probability the doctor must narrow down the possible list until a final diagnosis is reached.

As medicine is always changing, a competent doctor must try to keep up with new developments and be self-motivated to undertake continuing learning. This may be structured in lectures and conferences or unstructured based on daily reading and gaps in knowledge picked up when seeing patients. As a consequence of these demands a high level of accurate self-knowledge and honesty is required for professional practice together with a higher degree of self-motivation in a busy schedule.

In many cognitive disorders such as head injury or the early stages of Alzheimer's dementia, remote memories are relatively preserved but current and recent memories are substantially impaired (Kopelman, 1989). Consequently an affected individual may present with increasing problems in holding new information long enough to make a decision, and learning new material can be particularly difficult. There is an extensive literature on memory disorders within neuropsychology but surprisingly little work on memory impairment in doctors.

As we noted earlier, the term 'executive function' refers to the ability to plan, organise and prioritise activity. It also refers to mood regulation, motivation and self-discipline. When the frontal areas of the brain are damaged, the so-called 'dysexecutive syndrome' develops and the patient may become extremely apathetic and unable to decide what to do next. The doctor needs good executive abilities both to treat an individual patient, i.e. conduct a consultation, take a history, organise the information and treatment and to oversee a practice, office or department. Again there is an extensive literature on executive dysfunction but very little about the condition in doctors.

Aspects of cognition are also critical for the performance of psychomotor skills. For example, visuospatial skills are involved in a wide range of everyday activities and a doctor who becomes impaired cannot perform competently. A radiologist or histopathologist with a visual field defect and/or visual inattention, due perhaps to a cerebrovascular accident, may not be able to perceive stimuli in the hemispace contralateral to the lesion, and so may miss abnormalities without being aware of this difficulty.

Similarly the surgeon must remember the tasks involved in a number of operations, the order in which to perform them and must be skilled in physically performing these tasks. Surgeons must have particularly good visuospatial functioning and a high degree of fine motor control and co-ordination. If any one of these key areas of functioning is damaged, their performance is affected. There is now work being undertaken to look at surgical performance and it is possible using simulators and optical motion tracking to monitor dexterity and technical ability (Moorthy et al., 2003).

Examples of neurological disorders affecting neuropsychological function

This section aims to introduce some common conditions leading to a decline in cognitive functioning, namely, various types of dementia, alcoholic brain damage, head trauma, brain injury and depression. The ways these conditions can affect individuals are described and the potential implications in terms of deficiencies in the workplace are demonstrated by some examples in the section on head injuries.

Dementia

A key area of concern is the doctor with progressive dementia who may not be aware of increasing impairment. There are many causes of dementia (Galton & Hodges, 2003), which manifest with different symptoms and signs depending on the brain areas that may be involved and the stage of progression. Although considered to be a disease predominantly affecting older people, it can affect a younger age group. Dementia may also arise in the context of conditions such as multiple sclerosis, Parkinson's disease, epilepsy and a range of systemic disorders, including cardiovascular disease, vitamin deficiency and infection (e.g. HIV).

Alzheimer's dementia

Alzheimer's disease is the commonest cause of dementia and the average time period from diagnosis to death is about 10 years. However, rate of progression can vary between individuals. The time of onset can be difficult to pinpoint as the condition progresses very gradually. The cardinal symptom is virtually always memory impairment, accompanied by a deficit in naming and word-finding. As the disease progresses, the forgetfulness increases and there is reduced concentration, inflexibility in thinking and failure to solve problems and complete tasks. There may be lack of, or insufficient, insight into problems and the patient may overestimate their level of functioning. Progressively, patients may become very passive, inactive and unconcerned. There may appear to be signs of depression with low mood, emotional dullness, avoidance of social and stressful situations. There may also be the opposite effect, with disinhibited behaviour and inappropriate sexual or overemotional behaviour. In the later stages there is difficulty dressing and maintaining personal hygiene.

With increasing deterioration, verbal function declines with a reduced vocabulary and understanding of complex words and increasing word finding problems. There is a decline in visuospatial function and in a range of other cognitive skills. At a practical level this is demonstrated by not being able to use a map or getting lost in previously familiar surroundings and not being able to copy simple drawings.

The types of functional impairment in dementia are very closely related to the areas of the brain affected. This can be demonstrated by the differentiation of Alzheimer's disease from another type of dementia called 'fronto-temporal dementia'. In Alzheimer's dementia the medial temporal region is affected early, with cortical atrophy spreading to the parietal and temporal association areas and later to the frontal cortex and the brain stem nuclei. In fronto-temporal dementia, cortical atrophy occurs in the temporal and/or prefrontal cortex with the parietal and occipital lobes being spared – the relative degree of atrophy in the temporal and frontal lobes being very variable.

Fronto-temporal dementia

In fronto-temporal dementias, the mean age of onset is the mid-fifties and the mean duration of the disease is approximately 8 years, with a range of 2 to 17 years

(Gustafson, 2000). These dementias constitute a clinically heterogeneous group. Three variants have been identified:

1 frontal lobe degeneration, in which social behaviour and personality changes predominate
2 semantic dementia, in which a naming and word comprehension impairment predominates in the context of fluent speech; this is associated with left temporal degeneration, and with relative sparing of the hippocampi
3 progressive nonfluent aphasia, in which speech becomes very sparse, with phonological and syntactic errors; this is associated with left perisylvian atrophy.

In the frontal variant of fronto-temporal dementia, there are early changes in personality and behaviour and a decline in expressive speech. Behaviour is often disinhibited, tactless, flippant, indifferent and childish and leads to conflicts in the home and workplace. There is a greater lack of insight than in Alzheimer's disease. Personal hygiene and appearance deteriorate, with incontinence occurring quite early in the process. There may be overeating and excessive alcohol use. Eventually the patient becomes very apathetic and cannot decide what to do, with a marked reduction in spontaneous speech. In the temporal lobe variant of fronto-temporal dementia, there are either early problems with naming, word finding and verbal comprehension (semantic dementia) or a progressive (nonfluent) dysphasia.

Alcoholic brain damage

The medical profession is at high risk of alcohol abuse (Brooke, 1997). Even a moderate intake can impair memory, attention and other cognitive skills, including visuospatial processing, performance of complex tasks and decision making. The risk of road traffic accidents increases with increasing intake (Raynaud *et al.*, 2002). Alcohol and its metabolites are toxic to the brain and long-term high intake can lead to cerebral atrophy and enlarged ventricles. There is damage to the dorsolateral frontal and parietal regions. Binge drinkers seem to be less at risk of cognitive effects than daily heavy drinkers. Abstinence leads to an improvement and neuro-psychological research shows that some patients gradually improve over 3 to 5 years.

Head trauma and brain injury

Head trauma is common and can affect all ages especially after road traffic accidents. The level of damage can be unpredictable because the degree of cognitive impairment is not always related to the degree of physical damage. Quite severe and significant damage can occur in the absence of loss of consciousness or prolonged post-traumatic amnesia. An example is given below in Box 4.1. Outcomes from head injury are worse in older people who have been previously head injured, and in heavy drinkers, who have less brain function 'reserve'.

Even after a relatively mild head injury a post-concussion syndrome or post-traumatic stress disorder can develop. Patients complain of headache, dizziness, slower thinking and lack of concentration. They can have problems at work and experience fatigue. The syndrome often improves after 6 months but some patients are left with chronic symptoms and increased anxiety levels. Depression can develop at any time, but especially when patients realise they are not getting better as quickly as expected.

Moderate to severe head injuries can cause permanent damage. After acute treatment patients are frequently left with reduced mental processing speed, slowed reaction times, memory problems (involving both verbal and non-verbal material), speech and language difficulties, reduced attention span, difficulty with multi-tasking, decreased complex reasoning and impaired arithmetic skills.

Many of the changes in personality and behaviour are due to frontal lobe damage. In head trauma there is damage at two levels, the initial direct damage and the secondary damage due to acceleration/deceleration, which can be just as severe. The frontal and anterior temporal regions are particularly vulnerable to damage in head trauma. The frontal lobes are responsible for executive functioning: planning, motivation and decision making and mood regulation. In brain-injured patients there is often a very noticeable change to personality, which may involve apathy, disinterest, childishness, selfishness, impulsiveness, increased frustration, irritability and aggression. There may also be antisocial behaviour and sexual disinhibition. Major psychiatric symptoms are seen in approximately 25% of patients at 1 year. Social isolation may occur due to personality changes and lack of initiative, leading to further problems.

Improvement after brain injury is greatest in the first year and after this time improvement rate slows down. About a third of patients get back to previous employment, and rehabilitation can help to achieve this. They may often not be performing at the same level as before and may not cope at management levels, largely due to a decline in executive functioning. There is also a greater risk of depression and dementia in the longer term.

Below are some case histories from published sources which demonstrate the typical problems. The first and third are pilots and the second is a physician. The US Federal Aviation Administration (FAA) has issued guidance on assessment of head-injured aircrew and has high standards of fitness (Fiedler *et al.*, 2001). In the case of pilots, if these standards are not met then they may not be passed as fit to fly and have to be retrained, redeployed or retired on medical grounds.

Box 4.1

Case study: US Air Force pilot with minor head injury (Fiedler *et al.*, 2001)

A 34-year-old fighter pilot was playing a team ball game when the right temporal region of his head collided with another player's head. He completed the game but was confused and incoherent and could not remember what had happened in the game or recent life events. In hospital he had a minor abrasion and normal CT scan. His memory returned and he was discharged 8 hours later. The US Air Force has extremely strict fitness procedures and a doctor saw him 2 days after the accident. Although he had no physical symptoms he could not remember anything after the injury for $7\frac{1}{2}$ hours and was irritable. Within 6 weeks he had a full neuropsychological assessment and was found to have attention/concentration deficits and a lower IQ than previously in his pilot's tests. He was suspended from flying for 2 years after which he was re-evaluated and found to be closer to his premorbid state. He was then relicensed to fly. The current practice in the USAF now is to re-evaluate patients at 6 months.

Box 4.2

Case study: Physician in his 50s – 10 years after road traffic accident (Walsh, 1991)

The patient had been unconscious for 8 days after the accident. The brain damage resulted in uninhibited behaviour, double vision and anosmia (a common indicator of frontal lobe damage). He returned to work within a few weeks but appeared to have an altered personality leading to conflict with his partners in the practice and increased irritability and angry outbursts. He had previously been a diligent and easy-going person. He managed to continue his medical practice for 10 years, working alone with the help of his wife. Functional deficits appeared to be related to misinterpreting new information, inattention, forgetting names and arrangements and unpredictable behaviour. Formal neuropsychological testing revealed poor attention to complex instructions and difficulty solving complex and arithmetical problems. These findings indicated frontal lobe dysfunction and indeed a CT scan showed extensive damage to the frontal lobes. He seemed to have coped in the workplace because his wife had helped to organise his working life.

Box 4.3

Case study: A dangerous private pilot (Thieman, 2004)

A 45-year-old pilot was involved in an alcohol-related fight and suffered a right basilar skull fracture. An MRI confirmed contusions in the left temporal area and some intracerebral bleeding. He had aphasia and difficulty writing and was rehabilitated over a 3-month period. He had persistent speech and motor problems and little insight into his limitations. He also had a right visual field defect.

His job involved having to ferry aircraft for sale and, due to his expressive and receptive speech problems, it was felt that a return to work was unlikely.

Despite this he returned to flying and the FAA revoked his licence after he made errors thought to have resulted from his neurological condition. He still carried on flying and incurred serious infringements in procedures. Eventually the case went to court and an expert witness felt that his cognitive damage had led to his poor judgement and lack of insight into his impairments.

Depression

Depression can affect cognition but the difficulty often lies in deciding whether it is the actual depression itself that has caused the impairment or another underlying condition like dementia or brain trauma. In addition, medication can also affect cognition, for example, anticholinergic agents or steroids. The general view is that depression affects recent and current memory and learning processes. There is also a slowing of general mental functioning and deficits of executive function and attention (Austin *et al.*, 2001; Lezak, 1995).

Other causes of cognitive impairment include the effects of medication and recreational drug use and these are not covered in this review. Similarly, learning disabilities like dyslexia and dyscalculia may be due to brain dysfunction and necessitate highly specialised assessment and treatment, which are usually managed by educational psychologists and are not covered in this review.

Occupational health assessment

The occupational health physician may be the first person to see a doctor with cognitive problems. The patient may be referred for an opinion because of sickness absence, making errors, behaving in an inappropriate manner or not coping with routine tasks.

The main task of the physician is to determine whether the doctor is fit to work and whether any identifiable work or health factors are impacting on performance. The patient may need to be referred for more specialist assessment to a psychiatrist, occupational psychologist or neuropsychologist before definitive advice can be given.

The physician must take a full educational and job history so that previous levels of job functioning can be assessed. Any gaps in employment can be an indicator of health and performance problems and should be fully investigated if possible. Details of the current job and responsibilities should be documented, including working hours, workload, management structure, administrative support and potential litigation and complaints. The physician should explore with the patient any specific task-based problems and the level of insight into work problems. The referring organisation may have given very specific details of performance failures and workplace problems but if these are not available it is incumbent on the physician to investigate the failures and problems further and get as much information as possible. It may also be necessary to visit the workplace to gain an idea of the organisational environment and culture.

The physician must also obtain a full medical and social history and consider lifestyle factors like drugs and alcohol. If a personality or behavioural change is suspected then it may be necessary to obtain the patient's permission to speak to a partner or relative. The physician must also perform a very basic psychiatric and cognitive assessment. Traditionally, the Mini Mental State is used in these situations but it is not particularly sensitive and does not collect information on all potentially relevant areas of cognitive functioning.

An assessment at this stage can be quite simple, looking at orientation for time and place, memory of news events and personal history. Other relatively easy things to assess are naming of less common items, basic calculations, copying a clock face and basic designs, reading and writing, speech quality, repeating a sentence and some abstract thinking by interpretation of proverbs.

After an initial consultation the physician will usually have some idea whether there is a potentially significant problem which may need more investigation, together with input from other specialists. The key question is then whether the doctor is considered fit enough to continue working and in what capacity and with what reasonable adjustments and rehabilitation.

Neuropsychological and neuropsychiatric assessments

Clinical neuropsychology and neuropsychiatry are both concerned with relationships between abnormal brain function and behaviour, although there is an overlap between these two disciplines.

The neuropsychiatric contribution to assessment consists of taking a full psychiatric history (Kopelman, 1994a) and carrying out a full neurological and physical examination. The mental state is evaluated during the consultation, including the emotional consequences of brain disorders (e.g. depression, post-traumatic stress disorder), the presence of any psychotic syndrome or personality change, and a clinical ('screening') assessment of the cognitive state (Kopelman, 1994b). Further investigations are carried out including relevant blood tests, MRI or CT, EEG if required, and ECG, chest x-ray, or other neuro-imaging as required. Diagnosis and management take account of these findings as well as the results of the neuropsychological assessment.

Neuropsychology predominantly focuses on the analysis and quantification of cognitive impairments. A neuropsychological assessment contributes to the diagnosis of a brain disorder and localisation of lesion. Although the advent of neuro-imaging techniques has modified its role in terms of localisation, it still provides pertinent information in this regard, especially in the context of early dementia and relatively mild brain trauma, where structural imaging, including MRI, may not reveal abnormalities. Another role of a neuropsychological assessment is the differentiation between an organically based and a psychiatric disorder, for example between depression and mild dementia. Most importantly within the present context, it can provide unique information about an individual's functional abilities and the extent to which these are suited to specific occupations and responsibilities – these findings may also have implications for any cognitive rehabilitation.

There is no standard or universally accepted method of neuropsychological assessment. However, most clinicians commonly use techniques to identify a potential reduction in an individual's intellectual skills. These include abilities reflecting general knowledge and a wide range of problem-solving skills that may be cumulatively expressed with a single measure, referred to as 'IQ' (Intelligence Quotient). A reduction in a patient's IQ can be determined by comparing his/her performance on various intelligence tests with their pre-morbid or optimal IQ. The pre-morbid IQ may be estimated on the basis of educational and/or occupational backgrounds or, more objectively, on the basis of an individual's achievements on a specialised reading test, that is convertible to an IQ equivalent. The rationale for this procedure is that reading skill is relatively resistant to brain damage.

A deterioration in IQ does not provide guidance as to possible brain areas that may be dysfunctional/damaged. This is because each intelligence test involves multiple skills that are subserved by different parts of the brain. Moreover, lack of deterioration in IQ does not necessarily imply that a patient is cognitively intact. Patients may present with specific or 'focal' cognitive deficits that are known to be associated with damage in specific brain areas. Impairment in specific abilities, for instance in executive skills, may render people incapable of functioning properly in their everyday life or occupations. Consequently, in addition to the assessment of intellectual skills, a comprehensive neuropsychological assessment involves other tests that may reveal one or more focal deficits.

An important cognitive domain that is crucial to normal functioning is memory. Although the term 'memory' is commonly used as implying a unitary phenomenon, it comprises a range of skills that are dissociable, each having different anatomical correlates. These contrasting skills, for example, may be memory for verbal vs non-verbal material, short- vs long-term memory, ability to recall new information vs ability to recall distant past events. Other cognitive domains, such as language, object recognition, visuospatial and executive skills similarly comprise a range of multiple, independent processors that may be selectively preserved or impaired. For the identification of specific deficits in each cognitive domain, a range of tests should therefore be performed. All test results are compared to normative data according to an individual's age, taking into account that with the advancement of years, there is a natural reduction in an individual's efficiency, some cognitive skills being more affected than others. The correct interpretation of cognitive deficits helps the experienced clinician to make valid inferences that contribute to the diagnosis of a patient, including the differential diagnosis between organic and nonorganic disorders and between specific organically based disorders. This may be, for example, between Alzheimer's disease and vascular dementia or different Parkinsonian syndromes. This information is also of key importance in determining an individual's fitness to perform specific duties.

In the assessment of intellectual skills and specific cognitive deficits, it is important to consider and take account of a person's educational and cultural background and their physical and psychological state at the time of the assessment. Potential medication effects, such as those of anticholinergic drugs, also need to be considered since they are known to affect an individual's performance. There are ways that enable an examiner to carry out fairly comprehensive assessments of people who are not able to concentrate optimally for relatively long periods of time. In such circumstances, a clinician aims to sample a wide range of skills with brief procedures. Many of the published tests have been developed on white Anglo-American populations. Patient-tailored, including relatively culture-free tests, may also be administered to certain people who are not of white Anglo-American backgrounds, so that meaningful results can be obtained.

Remediability and intervention

Obviously, if a doctor has a treatable psychiatric condition which underlies or contributes to his/her cognitive impairment, treatment should be offered. For example, depression would be managed with an antidepressant and/or cognitive behaviour therapy. It is usual to reassess a client after treatment of the depression to see whether cognitive function has indeed returned to the expected premorbid level. Marital problems may require couple counselling, and conflict with colleagues may necessitate investigation and mediation. Problems with alcohol can be much more difficult to manage because of the risk of relapse, although a crisis at work may be the precipitant to successful abstinence. Clearly the factors precipitating and maintaining heavy drinking need to be explored and referral to an alcohol or substance misuse specialist may be required. Again, once the doctor has become abstinent, it will be appropriate to reassess cognitive function – although studies in heavy drinkers show that improvements following abstinence can gradually ac-cumulate over a matter of years. Rare cases of psychosis will need appropriate psychiatric intervention, and the risks of relapse need to be taken into account when planning for the future career. Personality change following frontal lobe damage can be much more intractable and difficult to manage – fitness to work needs to be assessed very carefully.

Similarly, treatable medical conditions need to be managed appropriately, such as in the case of Parkinson's disease. Newly diagnosed space-occupying lesions will need appropriate surgical intervention: more problematical may be decisions about the future career, once surgical and other cancer interventions have been com-pleted. Findings from the neuropsychological assessment will be particularly im-portant here. In the case of a dementia, anticholinesterase medications and memantine are available: their benefits are limited and, once a doctor has reached this stage, he/she is extremely unlikely to be fit to practise. In cerebro-vascular disorders, the most important aspect of management consists of minimalising the risk of further vascular episodes with anti-hypertensive agents, statins, aspirin, encouragement to give up cigarettes or alcohol, etc. Again, the neuropsychological assessment is critical: a doctor may be able to practise after a relatively minor cerebro-vascular episode, but more generalised vascular changes will make him/her unfit to practise. Medical intervention in head injury depends on the specific requirements of the patient, but the most important factor in recovery is time, and repeated neuropsychological assessments may be required to make the decision as to whether the victim is fit to return to practise.

Referral to a rehabilitation unit may well be appropriate, particularly in head injury, as the doctor may benefit from psychological and occupational therapy interventions. These vary from part-time outpatient programmes to full-time inpatient centres. Psychological strategies for coping with memory disorders in-clude the use of external aids, such as computers, a diary, a pager system, etc., or the use of 'internal' strategies to improve memory, e.g. errorless learning, the use of mnemonics (Wilson, 1999; Kapur, Glisky & Wilson, 2002). Such strategies may be helpful to a practising doctor with relatively minor cognitive impairments (Evans, 2003). Those with more severe impairments may benefit from such rehabilitation, but they are unlikely to return to work.

Conclusion

Where there is an actual or suspected cognitive impairment in a doctor, neuro-psychiatric and neuropsychological assessments, as well as an occupational health assessment, are obviously essential. From the above, it will be seen that such assessments can be complex and multidimensional as cognitive functioning is affected by such a wide range of factors and a variety of medical and psychiatric disorders. In general, assessment will need to be carried out by relevant experts, as many doctors and even occupational psychologists are not expert in assessing what get called 'higher functions'. No quick questionnaire is available to perform this task, and it is very unlikely that it would be possible to construct such a test. Moreover, it needs to be emphasised that, to date, occupational medicine and occupational psychology, on the one hand, and neuropsychiatry/neuropsychology, on the other, have been developed and researched by very different groups of people, and there has been very little interaction between them. The application of neuropsychiatry/neuropsychology to the workplace is an important topic for future research.

Further reading

For further reading about cognitive/neuropsychological abnormalities please refer to *Neuropsychological Assessment* (Lezak, 1995), the *New Oxford Textbook of Psychiatry* (Gelder *et al.*, 2000), the *Oxford Handbook of Clinical Neuropsychology* (Halligan, Kischka & Marshall, 2003) and the *Handbook of Memory Disorders* (Baddeley *et al.*, 2002).

References

Austin MP, Mitchell P and Goodwin GM (2001) Cognitive deficits in depression: possible implications for functional neuropathology. *British Journal of Psychiatry.* **178**: 200–6.

Baddeley AD, Kopelman MD and Wilson BA (eds) (2002) *The Handbook of Memory Disorders* (2e). John Wiley & Sons, Chichester.

Brooke D (1997) Impairment in the medical and legal professions. *J Psychosomatic Research.* **43**(1): 27–34.

Evans JJ (2003) Rehabilitation of executive deficits. In: BA Wilson (ed.) *Neuropsychological Rehabilitation: theory and practice.* Swets and Zeitlinger Publishers, Netherlands, p. 58.

Fiedler E *et al.* (2001) *Assessment of Head-injured Aircrew: comparison of FAA and USAF procedures. DOT/FAA/AM-01/11.* Federal Aviation Administration, Washington, DC. Available at: www.hf.faa.gov/docs/508/docs/cami/0111.pdf [Accessed 20 September 2004].

Galton CJ and Hodges JR (2003) Alzheimer's disease and other dementias. In: DA Warrell, TM Cox and JD Firth (eds) *Oxford Textbook of Medicine* (4e). Oxford University Press, Oxford, pp. 1034–45.

Gelder MG, López-Ibor JJ Jr and Andreasen NC (eds) (2000) *New Oxford Textbook of Psychiatry.* Oxford University Press, Oxford.

General Medical Council (2001) *Good Medical Practice* [online] (3e). General Medical Council, London. Available at: www.gmc-uk.org/standards/default.htm [Accessed 22 September 2004].

Gustafson L (2000) Frontotemporal dementias. In: MG Gelder, JJ López-Ibor Jr and NC Andreasen (eds) *New Oxford Textbook of Psychiatry.* Oxford University Press, Oxford, p. 398.

Halligan PW, Kischka U and Marshall JC (eds) (2003) *Handbook of Clinical Neuropsychology.* Oxford University Press, Oxford.

Joint Aviation Authorities. *JAR-FLC1 Flight Crew Licensing (Aeroplane)* [online]. Joint Aviation Authorities, Hoofddorp. JAR documents available at: www.jaa.nl. [Accessed 15 August 2005].

Kapur N, Glisky EL and Wilson BA (2002) External memory aids and computers in memory rehabilitation. In: AD Baddeley, MD Kopelman and BA Wilson (eds) *The Handbook of Memory Disorders* (2e). John Wiley & Sons, Chichester, pp. 757–83.

Kopelman MD (1989) Remote and autobiographical memory, temporary cortex memory and frontal atrophy in Korsakoff and Alzheimer patients. *Neuropsychologia.* **27**(4): 437–60.

Kopelman MD (1994a) Structured psychiatric interview: psychiatric history and assessment of the mental state. *British Journal of Hospital Medicine.* **52**(2–3): 93–8.

Kopelman MD (1994b) Structured psychiatric interview: assessment of the cognitive state. *British Journal of Hospital Medicine*. **52**(6): 277–81.

Lezak MD (1995) *Neuropsychological Assessment* (3e). Oxford University Press, New York.

Moorthy K *et al.* (2003) Objective assessment of technical skills in surgery. *BMJ*. **327**(7422): 1032–7.

Raynaud M *et al.* (2002) Alcohol is the main factor in excess traffic accident fatalities in France. *Alcoholism, Clinical and Experimental Research*. **26**(12): 1833–9.

Thieman PW. *Brain Injury and Flying: 'scary'*. Federal Surgeon's Medical Bulletin [online]. Federal Aviation Administration, Washington, DC. Available at: www.faa.gov/avr/aam/fasb597/archtoc.htm [Accessed 20 September 2004].

Turnbull J *et al.* (2000) Cognitive difficulty in physicians. *Academic Medicine*. **75**(2): 177–181.

Walsh KW (1991) *Understanding Brain Damage* (2e). Churchill Livingstone, Edinburgh, New York.

Wilson BA (1999) *Case Studies in Neuropsychological Rehabilitation*. Oxford University Press, Oxford.

Chapter 5

Are psychological factors linked to performance?*

Jenny Firth-Cozens and Jennifer King

The main thrust of recent work towards safer, higher quality healthcare emphasises the importance of organisational systems, taking its lead from other industries such as aviation (Sexton, Thomas & Helmreich, 2000). Nevertheless, healthcare differs from other areas in that the relationship between the clinician and the patient has been shown to affect aspects of process and outcome. For example, just as findings from other types of organisations show that dissatisfied staff lead to dissatisfied customers (Schneider & Bowen, 1985), so too within healthcare there are studies which show that the quality of patient care, such as their general adherence to treatment (DiMatteo *et al.*, 1993) and no-show rates (Linn *et al.*, 1985), are related to physician and patient satisfaction.

These areas of literature demonstrate that individual aspects of the clinicians affect the doctor-patient relationship and are likely to have an indirect effect on outcomes. Their mental health will be one aspect of this (discussed in Chapter 2), as will be their personality and attitudes discussed below. In fact, many studies now suggest that aspects of the individuals, such as general dissatisfaction, are probably dispositional, are certainly long-lasting despite life changes, and make an important contribution to perception of the workplace, to stress, and so possibly to the quality of the work produced (Costa, McCrae & Zonderman, 1987). While some actions of the individual that lead to poor care will be due to a lack of knowledge or training, others are to do with personality or attitudes, leading to poor interactions with patients or other staff, poor leadership skills, or to a greater likelihood of providing care which is less safe or of lower quality.

These individual factors and their potential or actual relationship to patient care have rarely been investigated within medicine. However, there are numerous studies which look in particular at the force of different types of personality and attitudes on particular behaviours which are highly relevant to medicine. This chapter will consider the potential effects of different types of personality, and different attitudes, on medical performance, including safety and interpersonal relationships. It uses primarily literature from management, military, social and health psychology fields, but also reviews studies from medicine and other health professions.

---

* Part of this review is based on a paper by Firth-Cozens, Cording & Ginsburg in *Quality & Safety in Health Care*, 2003.

What are the psychological factors that influence doctors' performance?

Attitudes

It is generally accepted within organisations and across industries, particularly those which are high risk, that staff need appropriate attitudes to enable safe, thoughtful care to take place. This has been demonstrated on the individual level in the aviation industry where a series of studies showed links between attitude and performance in terms of aircraft management and safety. The pilots had some time previously completed safety attitude measures and were later independently rated as pilots along a scale from 'outstanding' to 'extremely poor' (Helmreich et al., 1986). Comparing the attitudes of those being scored at these two extremes, the study found that they differed most significantly in the following:

- My decision-making ability is as good in emergencies as in routine flying situations (superior – disagree).
- Captains should encourage their First Officers to question procedures during normal flight operations and in emergencies (superior – agree).
- Pilots should be aware of and sensitive to the personal problems of fellow crew members (superior – agree).
- There are no circumstances (except total incapacitation) where the First Officer should assume command of the aircraft (superior – disagree).

These results show that being the type of person who wants total control, who feels invincible, and who is probably a poor team player, makes the worst pilot. The authors talk of the 'macho' pilot, the one who 'does not recognize personal limitations due to stress and emergencies, does not utilize the resources of fellow crew members, is less sensitive to problems and reactions of others, and tends to employ a consistent, authoritarian style of management' (Helmreich et al., 1986: 1200).

In terms of ability to change, the authors later showed that crew resource management training changed these attitudes appropriately for most pilots (Helmreich & Wilhelm, 1991). However, the attitudes of one group actually became less appropriate over the course. Those pilots who were low in both autocratic traits and expressive interpersonal characteristics, as well as being poor in performance, actually developed worse attitudes. The authors nicknamed them the 'no stuff', as opposed to the 'right stuff' (interpersonally good, not autocratic, and high performers) and the 'wrong stuff' (those who were autocratic but performed well), both of whom changed their attitudes still further for the better. They conclude that this has the worrying implication that 'the types of individuals who seem to need the training most may be less likely to be influenced in the desired manner' (Helmreich & Wilhelm, 1991: 298). These results very much show the importance of different leadership styles for safety and quality but also that, for most people, they can be changed for the better (Firth-Cozens & Mowbray, 2001).

Despite these findings, the relationship between an individual's attitudes and his or her performance is by no means clear (Schaper, 2002). People can learn to behave in ways which are appropriate (such as police learning not to arrest young black men with no obvious cause), but still retain the same attitudes (such as racism). Although findings vary at this individual level, there is nevertheless evidence that attitudes can also affect performance at the organisational level. For example, Ostroff surveyed over 13 000 school teachers and found that job satisfaction along with their attitudes in terms of their commitment, adjustment and psychological stress were predictive of school performance (Ostroff, 1992).

The problem with the loose term of 'attitudes' is that the meaning changes with each study, as the Ostroff study shows. Nevertheless, the findings from the Helmreich studies show that sensible measures of attitudes about safety might be important in terms of predicting who may be less safe in healthcare, particularly as they correspond with other research findings in areas such as leadership and safety. A very early study looked at the values and attitudes of medical students in relation to preferred career choice (Linn & Zeppa, 1982). They found that those choosing particular forms of surgery were more cynical and authoritarian than those selecting general surgery, but the latter had higher self-esteem. All those choosing surgery had higher tolerance of ambiguity than other students. Although none of the values or attitudes related to their grades, they did relate to ward behaviour as judged by house staff and academic staff. Students who valued academic achievement more and independence less, and those who were less authoritarian with higher ego strength, were classed as better ward performers. The authors questioned whether this might be because the judgement of those rating ward performance was affected in turn by these authoritarian, independent attitudes. However, they do match the Helmreich findings with pilots described above as well as those of good and bad leaders described elsewhere (Firth-Cozens & Mowbray, 2001).

Personality

The Big Five personality factors

The Five Factor Model of Personality, widely known as the Big Five, is the most intensively researched model in the field of personality and is a reliable predictor of job performance in a wide variety of occupations (Barrick & Mount, 1991; Barrick, Mount & Judge, 2001). Its five factors are Extraversion, Agreeableness, Emotional Stability, Openness and Conscientiousness, with the latter being the most consistently valid predictor across performance measures in all occupations studied.

The Big Five personality factors

- **Conscientiousness:** being hardworking, organised and self-disciplined.
- **Emotional Stability:** being resilient and relaxed under pressure.
- **Openness:** being creative, open to change, intellectually curious.
- **Extraversion:** being outgoing.
- **Agreeableness:** being co-operative.

Emotional Stability (resilience under pressure) was also found to be a generalisable predictor of overall work performance. Emotional Stability is defined by lack of anxiety, hostility, depression and personal insecurity. Extraversion (sociability, dominance, ambition, excitement seeking, positive emotions) has been found to be related to job performance in occupations where interactions with others are a significant part of the job (for example, sales and management, but is also clearly relevant in most areas of medicine). There is somewhat more limited evidence that shows that higher scores on Extraversion are associated with greater training proficiency, possibly because extraverted trainees are more active during training and ask more questions (Barrick, Mount & Judge, 2001).

The Big Five trait of Openness informs our understanding of how receptive an individual will be to learning and change. It appears that employees who are intellectual, curious, imaginative and have broader interests may be more likely to benefit from training. Adaptability has also been noted as an important behavioural marker for successful surgical outcomes (Carthey *et al.*, 2003).

Characteristics of Type A personality

People who are more aggressive, competitive and impatient are more likely to fall into the personality category of Type A, which has been recognised since the 1950s as a predictor of increased risk of coronary heart disease. It is the heightened hostility that this type of person shows which has subsequently been found to be the most predictive of CHD. However, Type A and Type B individuals also show differences in various vocational activities and performances (Waldron *et al.*, 1980), and those who are Type As have more traffic accidents, greater frequency of breaking traffic laws, higher impatience when driving, more aggression on the road and more risky driving behaviours (Perry & Baldwin, 2000). Such behavioural outcomes – accidents, law-breaking etc. – may translate well into the world of medicine. The forceful, confident Type A is highly rewarded in the modern world – presumably also within medicine, nursing and management – and therefore an area for future research would be to discover the extent to which their safety record (or that of their organisation) matches that of Type B people. In terms of adaptability, it has been shown to be very difficult to change Type A behaviours, presumably because within the workplace they are often so rewarded.

Self-criticism and self-esteem

There are a number of characteristics which show a U-shaped curve in terms of performance: too much or too little is likely to be problematic, and the optimum is around the centre. In terms of self-criticism, for example, high self-criticism is related to depression in doctors and predictive of the condition over many years; it is clearly not a healthy characteristic for doctors (Firth-Cozens, 1997). Blatt (Blatt & Zuroff, 1992) describes the pattern as 'characterised by self-criticism and feelings of unworthiness, inferiority, failure, and guilt. These individuals engage in constant harsh self-scrutiny and evaluation and have a chronic fear of being disapproved of and criticised ... They strive for excessive achievement and perfection, are often highly competitive and work hard ...'

On the other hand, those with particularly low self-criticism have more problems with colleagues and with patients (Firth-Cozens, 1985). Getting a balance of responsibility – not blaming yourself (or others) for everything that goes wrong and being able to take the credit for things that go well – is a form of cognitive restructuring which could be taught in medical school in courses on error and risk management (Brewin & Firth-Cozens, 1997).

Similarly, in studies outside medicine, high self-esteem has frequently been linked to aggression (Papps & O'Carroll, 1998). This is now seen as a reflection not so much of high confidence and self-worth as of an underlying insecurity which leads to more grandiose, narcissistic behaviours which, when threatened, can cause aggression (Salmivalli, 2001). Aggression is unlikely to help effective teamwork and safety, and so the type of self-image which gives rise to aggressive behaviours is again an aspect of the individual worth considering in terms of patient care.

Finally, confidence is seen as a good thing in a doctor and to some extent medical students are chosen for their confidence which is likely to be valuable in their dealings with patients and with colleagues. However, like self-criticism and self-esteem, it is likely that there is a U-shaped curve here too – too much or too little confidence is going to be problematic in medicine and other work. In fact, these characteristics – confidence, self-esteem and low self-criticism – may well be so highly related that their division is confusing rather than helpful. Nevertheless, in terms of change, it is likely that high self-criticism may be more susceptible to cognitive restructuring, while the rather more grandiose core of low self-criticism, high confidence and high self-esteem may require more traditional psychodynamic interventions. However, this is a clinical judgement not yet based on evidence.

The extent to which narcissistic behaviour can be changed is controversial. There is a view that no known therapy is effective with narcissism itself (Millon & Davis, 2000), though some therapies are reasonably successful in terms of coping with some of its effects. Later in this chapter we outline the management literature regarding the ability to change related work-based behaviours.

Perfectionism

From a patient's point of view, having a doctor who is a perfectionist sounds like good news. However, taken to its extreme, the doctor may slip into obsessional-compulsive behaviour patterns, checking and re-checking signs and symptoms, for example, and finding it difficult to make decisions. Perfectionism also correlates with depression, anxiety, eating disorders and other mental health problems. Hewitt and others (2003) and Flett & Hewitt (2002) argue that the self-oriented perfectionist – one with an internally motivated desire to be perfect – has a vulnerability for psychological disorders. Self-oriented perfectionists cope well in situations of low stress but, they argue, are more likely to become depressed or anxious in high-stress situations. In this way it is likely that high perfectionism is very similar to high self-criticism. In the UK, O'Connor and O'Connor (2003) have found that hopelessness and general distress can be predicted by an interaction between perfectionism and avoidance/coping, but not by perfectionism alone. If people have good coping skills, perfectionism is not damaging.

Remediation is therefore most likely to be successful if good coping skills are taught and if cognitive strategies are used to challenge perfectionism. However, Flett and Hewitt (2002) do not focus on lowering high personal standards – which might be a traditional cognitive approach – but on exploring the precursors to perfectionism such as the need to be accepted and cared for.

The risky personality

Taking risks is likely to be an inevitable part of some fields of medicine, in particular surgery. It may be more important that a clinician is able to recognise that he or she is actually doing something risky.

A widely based literature search has resulted in only one example of assessing the relationship between personality and healthcare risk (Rabaud *et al.*, 2000). However, there is a very large and relevant literature from the areas of health psychology and social psychology looking at both risk perception and personality factors linked to risk taking. Although a few studies involve risky workplaces such as Antarctica (Burns & Sullivan, 2000), most focus on groups such as those who do extreme sports or who take part in unsafe sex, or who are criminals, gamblers or drug-takers. In these studies, not surprisingly, risk taking has been seen as a bad thing, leading to poor outcomes. However, sometimes having an ability to take risks can be a positive attribute depending on the context: for example, a meta-analysis (Stewart & Roth, 2001) has shown entrepreneurs to have an appropriately higher risk-taking propensity than managers. Even in healthcare, it has not necessarily been seen negatively; for example, one study examines nurses who become managers and who may not have sufficient risk propensity to deliver services more intensely, faster, and at lower cost (Smith & Friedland, 1998).

Most studies focus on the negative aspects of risk propensity, and it is this area which has implications for patient safety. The first research area to consider is risk perception – the fact that some people can see danger more easily than others. This is an important part of healthcare since, if a doctor or nurse is able to see risk, then it is likely that he or she is more likely to do something to avoid it. One way to encourage greater risk perception is to increase mental readiness (McDonald, Orlick & Letts, 1995), to visualise each case – for example, each operation – beforehand so as to anticipate every risk which might arise and how these can be tackled. High Reliability Organisations (HROs) use this method of anticipating and planning for future surprises to help create safe scenarios (Rochlin, 1999). Research shows that some of our best surgeons appear to do this (McDonald, Orlick & Letts, 1995; Carthey *et al.*, 2003) and there is no reason why this ability cannot be taught.

Just because people can see risk, it does not necessarily follow that they will avoid it. Some people are positively attracted to risky activities and actions. The association between being able to perceive risk and changing one's behaviour accordingly is not so clear-cut (Burns & Sullivan, 2000). Similarly, others may believe, with unrealistic faith, in the protection and infallibility of their safety systems. Studies of coping strategies have shown optimistic faith to be good for one's mental health, but it may be that a certain level of pessimism is necessary for delivering good healthcare. Risk perception increases dramatically once people sustain a major incident: for example, after the destruction of some towns by Hurricane Hugo, huge precautions were put in place by those who had been hit in order to prevent future damage on that scale. However, the towns nearby which the hurricane by chance barely missed were much less likely to make changes (Norris, Smith & Kaniasty, 1999): their risk perception remained low. Even if objective data on hazards, such as reports of death or disability, are given, studies show that strongly held views on risk levels are actually quite resistant to change (Slovic, 1987). We do learn from our errors and experiences (rather than from data alone), but we may not always learn the right things; so various forms of defensive medicine may arise from the experience of being sued or complained against, while a death from an early discharge from hospital may lead to a doctor always keeping patients in hospital too long.

If people are still attracted to the risks they see, then their behaviour falls within the area of the risky personality known as sensation-seeking. The concept of sensation-seeking includes factors of disinhibition, thrill- and adventure-seeking, impulsivity, boredom susceptibility, sociability and aggression, depending upon the measure. For example, a study of adolescents found that risk-seeking (including disinhibition, a sense of invulnerability, experience-seeking, boredom susceptibility and thrill-seeking) predicted delinquent behaviours of alcohol abuse and risky driving (Greene *et al.*, 2000). Within healthcare, someone with this psychological make-up may simply choose an area of work where the dangers are higher, and be satisfied by the thrill this provides. This type of personality may choose dangerous procedures, or generally deliver less safe care, in order to find their stimulation. As stated earlier, research on this topic within healthcare is almost non-existent, but the evidence from elsewhere suggests that it may be an important area to pursue since there is a growing body of studies across decades and across continents which strongly suggests that 'sensation-seeking' and related drives or characteristics lead to a variety of dangerous behaviours such as gambling, drug and alcohol abuse, speeding, extreme sports and violence (Zuckerman & Kuhlman, 2000). Again, it is undoubtedly true that these extreme behaviours appear also in healthcare staff, or translate into other forms of unacceptable risk within the workplace.

High sensation-seekers tend to *perceive* risk as lower than low sensation-seekers and anticipate less anxiety when they are in the situation (Horvath & Zuckerman, 1993; Merrill *et al.*, 1994). Sensation-seeking has been shown to be linked to biochemical processes (Bardo, Donohew & Harrington, 1996), but cognitive processes also have a role in influencing decisions (Pinkerton & Abramson, 1995) and cognitions are likely to be a more useful target for change, perhaps being tackled in similar ways to addiction problems. There is evidence too that sensation-seeking may be used to compensate for anhedonia, or lower mood: it may be that helping people to tackle these aspects of their make-up would be useful. However, this is likely to require individual cognitive-behavioural therapy or other psychotherapy.

Only one study has emerged which explored the potential link between a risky personality and unsafe healthcare practices (Rabaud *et al.*, 2000). Using the Zuckerman sensation-seeking scales as one of several potential predictors of risky behaviour in nurses, the study found that risky practices were best predicted by a mixture of individual characteristics, including a low threshold for boredom, along with traditional job-related factors such as being less experienced and having a permanent position, meaning perhaps that you are less likely to see the risk of unemployment. Sensation-seeking seems to be a characteristic well worth further investigation in terms of its potential effects on the quality of care provided as well as the fact that other behaviours, such as drinking and drug use, are greater in those who are high on this factor.

In our literature review, no evidence was found to suggest that sensation-seeking can be changed, though investigating the factors that might lead to it, including the cognitive predictors (Pinkerton & Abramson, 1995), might help the design of an intervention. There is also evidence that it is affected by context, and contexts can also be changed – sometimes more easily than individuals. For example, alcohol abuse is influenced by sensation-seeking characteristics in 'boring' situations (Hoyle, 2000). Similarly, impulsiveness, clumsiness and lower mood rise with sleep loss (Sicard, Jouve & Blin, 2001), suggesting that sleep loss may increase risky behaviours as it lowers cognitive ability and dexterity (Firth-Cozens & Cording, 2004).

Different career paths might also interact with some personalities and psychological states to produce higher dissatisfaction which in turn may affect care (Firth-Cozens, Lema & Firth, 1999).

Personality type

Type, as outlined by the Myers Briggs Type Indicator® (MBTI), is described in a number of books (e.g. Firth-Cozens, Lema & Firth, 1999; Kroeger & Thuesen, 1989) and is the most-used psychological test in organisations worldwide. Type theory is based on the idea that an individual has characteristics and preferences that make up one of 16 types (*see* Table 5.1). Type clearly has major implications for behaviour and performance in medicine. For example, those high on the dimension of intuition might be inclined to ignore detail, while on the other side, those high on sensing might become too absorbed with test results and ignore the bigger picture. People who are more judging might be organised, but may rush to a diagnosis too soon, while those high on perceiving might find it more difficult to make a final decision. The dimension which causes the most difficulties among colleagues is the thinking–feeling dimension. Thinkers are prone to being somewhat blunt and critical, making decisions according to logic and rationality and justice. Feelers may be seen as rather emotionally demanding, needing appreciation and making decisions on interpersonal issues and values (*see* Table 5.1).

Table 5.1 The Myers Briggs Type Indicator® (MBTI) dimensions

Extraverts (E): Get your strength from being with others; where people know a lot about you quickly and you are likely to talk first, think later. You may be more perceptive of things around you.	**Introverts (I):** Where you like your private time for yourself; prefer to think about things before saying them, but like stating them without interruption. People may miss your meaning or ideas as they are not always expressed.
Sensors (S): Concentrate on the moment rather than the future, and would rather do something than think about it; prefer jobs with tangible results, and get frustrated over 'waffle'.	**Intuitives (N):** Tend to think about several things at once, often future-focused rather than the present; dislike 'boring detail'; enjoy looking for connections behind things; give general instructions and can't understand why people push you for specifics.
Thinkers (T): Stay cool, logical and objective; settle disputes on what is just and fair; don't mind making difficult decisions involving people as you think it's better to be truthful than liked.	**Feelers (F):** Like to take people's feelings into account when making decisions; try to meet people's needs and ask 'How will this affect them?'; hate conflict; and are seen as taking things too personally sometimes.
Judgers (J): Have a right place for everything and have your days well organised – and long for others to be the same; like to get things done and out of the way, sometimes too quickly.	**Perceivers (P):** Are easily distracted and casual about deadlines; are often accused of being disorganised, but believe that spontaneity is better than neatness; change the topic often when you talk (especially if also an N); don't like to be pinned down.

Clack's studies, using the MBTI on London doctors (Clack *et al.*, 2004), show that male doctors (and a higher proportion of women doctors than in the general population) in her sample are predominantly Ts, while nurses are predominantly Fs. Although none of these characteristics is seen as carved in stone, and is only a preference for behaviour, they nevertheless have great implications for interpersonal relationships as well as the way people work together. Moreover, she found that type differences affected their communications with patients too, and this has implications for communications training in medicine. Undoubtedly some of the accusations of bullying which are increasing in medicine could be explained by T–F conflicts (Paice & Firth-Cozens, 2003). Teaching about these various types and the usefulness of differences in teams would help young doctors to recognise their own behaviours and the effects these may have on those who are not like them. This understanding and recognition also has implications for how one can modify one's behaviour.

Personality factors that can predict failure

There is a growing literature in the management field that seeks to identify the personality factors that are associated with performance failure in individuals who have reached senior (leadership) positions. This research is potentially highly relevant to doctors in helping us understand how they 'derail', that is, doctors whose health, conduct or performance subsequently puts their employment or registration into question. The original research on management derailment was conducted on failed Sears executives (Bentz, 1985). It identified seven themes associated with performance failure:

- being unable to delegate or prioritise
- being reactive rather than proactive
- being unable to maintain relationships with an extended network of contacts
- being unable to build a team
- having poor judgement
- being a slow learner and
- having an 'overriding personality defect'.

Research by McCall and Lombardo (1983) and later research at the Center for Creative Leadership replicated and refined Bentz's findings. Leslie and Van Velsor (1997) summarised this research in terms of four themes related to performance failure:

1 problems with interpersonal relationships (e.g. being aloof, cold, arrogant)
2 failure to meet business objectives (betraying trust, not following through, overly ambitious)
3 inability to build or lead a team
4 inability to change or adapt to a transition (not strategic, conflict with upper management).

These themes were enduring over time and across countries, emerging as consistent findings from a large number of studies on derailment.

These executives, whilst in post, were often viewed as technical geniuses or tenacious problem-solvers. But as the demands of their job became greater, their early strengths became weaknesses and began to matter. There are some strong potential parallels with doctors. Medical training has a strong emphasis on the technical skills, but the transition to consultant or principal in general practice requires a much more complex range of interpersonal and management skills. Doctors are particularly vulnerable during and shortly after these transitions to a leadership role, often with little training or insight into what this role requires. Medical students making the transition to becoming a doctor are similarly vulnerable. The stress and pressure of these additional responsibilities may trigger self-defeating characteristics.

Hogan and Hogan (1997) developed an inventory to assess the dysfunctional attributes of employed adults with a view to identifying characteristics that underlie career derailment and to show how these characteristics impede leadership effectiveness. Hogan's research, based on the DSM-IV classification of personality disorders, identified three main factors, described as the tendencies to 'blow up, show off or conform' when under pressure. These correspond with and are based on Horney's original distinction between three types of behaviour under pressure: moving against, moving away and moving towards (Horney, 1950). This led to the development of a psychometric tool, the Hogan Development Survey (HDS), for use in occupational, rather than clinical, settings, which can identify these self-defeating characteristics. This is a tool with great potential for diagnosing some of the behaviours that may be contributing to derailment in doctors.

Hogan's work is useful because it focuses on the *behaviours* that get doctors into trouble, which may often be remediable, rather than the reasons behind these behaviours, which may be less easily remedied. In particular Hogan highlights the concept of 'overplayed strengths'. This is a more constructive route to remediation because it potentially encourages a focus on strength rather than weakness – helping the doctor to recognise where a particular behaviour can be helpful in certain situations, but a problem in others. This has similarities with the MBTI characteristics where each dimension is seen as producing positive aspects of behaviour unless used to extremes.

Can derailment be prevented? Leslie and Van Velsor (1997) argue that simply moving to a different organisation does not always prevent further problems since the critical factors stem from interpersonal skills and ability to adapt, rather than from the norms and values of the organisation. In order to change, the person needs to be willing, and supported, to work on some relatively tough development issues – including self-esteem and the need for control. Understanding why it may be difficult to relate comfortably to others, to be able to learn in the face of change or to be able to let go of the need for personal achievement in order to develop the team may involve facing issues about trust, security or need for power. These are insights usually associated with good psychotherapy since the learning that results from such insights often involves a high degree of emotional investment.

Leslie and Van Velsor argue that derailment is a useful lens through which to view and understand the leadership role as it can bring to the surface some important issues about organisational demands and the ways in which people are responding to change. They highlight the wealth of studies that show that not being able to learn from experience is a major, if not the major, factor in derailing careers.

Can psychological factors and their impact be assessed?

Psychological testing in medicine

A psychological test is essentially 'an objective and standardised measure of a sample of behaviour' (Anastasi and Urbin, 1997).

Unlike other industries, healthcare has rarely made use of psychometrics for selection purposes, except with its managers. Where measurement psychometrics have been used it has been remarkably successful, outranking all other factors in predicting some aspects of job performance (Reeve, Vickers & Horton, 1993). A study using one particular measure of personality – Cattell's 16PF plus interview with 62 training anaesthetists – followed them for 3–8 years, looking at academic, clinical, behavioural and overall performance (Hunter & Hunter, 1984). Performance was best predicted by the positive ends of the 16PF scales of dull/bright, unstable/stable, timid/socially bold and casual/controlled, and by scores in the middle of the scales of detached/warmhearted, expedient/conscientious and relaxed/tense. Gough and Bradley have also reported similar results for the 16PF with anaesthetists in the USA (Gough, Bradley & McDonald, 1991). These studies indicate that the 16PF may be a very useful tool in terms of personality and performance, but future studies should consider its use and long-term power in predicting performance in other specialties. It is interesting that, despite such positive and useful results, this form of selection remains so rare.

A number of studies have looked at the characteristics necessary for a good surgeon. Spatial reasoning has come out as the most important (Stevenson & Henley, 1989; Gibbons, Gudas & Gibbons, 1983) along with verbal reasoning in terms of communications skills, while another study suggests that trainers of future surgeons should be developing their higher-order cognitive skills such as problem solving and justification of actions (Hall, Ellis & Hamdorf, 2003). One study which begins to overcome these problems looked at behavioural markers of surgical excellence (Carthey *et al.*, 2003). The markers they reported were those found useful in aviation: technical skill, mental readiness and resilience, cognitive flexibility, anticipation, situational awareness and safety awareness, alongside team and organisational factors. Flexibility and resilience map onto the Big Five factors of Openness and Emotional Stability, respectively. Behaviours come from cognitions which are themselves strongly influenced by mental state and disposition. Behaviours and cognitions may be easier to recognise and to change than aspects of a person's disposition. In addition, research such as this focuses on the positive as much as the negative: what it takes to make an excellent surgeon (adaptability and good communication skills, for example) is just as important.

The problem with all these studies is, first, that different outcome measures are used between studies and, second, that such a variety of potential predictors are found useful. Future research should use the strongest of these studies in terms of design and replication, and the strongest findings (such as those using the 16PF or the Big Five), to form the basis of a longitudinal study of personality and skills across different medical specialties. Outcome measures require good face and concurrent validity in terms of patient care. This is expensive research with no quick answers, but without doing it, medical selection will remain considerably behind other professions and industries.

Integrity testing and 'counterproductive' work behaviours

Integrity is crucial in medicine and has also been shown to be an important factor in demonstrating trustworthiness in leaders as well (*see* Chapter 9). Integrity tests, shown to be reliable in a meta-analytic study (Ones, Viswesvaran & Schmidt, 1993), are used in job selection to help screen out potentially dishonest employees or those with counterproductive work behaviours (CWB). They measure such constructs as honesty, delinquency, conscientiousness and reliability. A related area of research considers aspects of the environment or work situation that may predict CWB (for example, workplace stressors such as noise, overcrowding, extreme temperatures; social characteristics such as work group norms).

Measures of counterproductive tendencies (the personality traits underlying counterproductive behaviours) have been divided into two categories: overt integrity tests and personality-based measures. The primary purpose of overt integrity tests has been to predict theft at work and other illegal or dishonest behaviour. Personality-based integrity tests have been developed to predict CWB including theft but also general dishonesty, laziness, aggression, disruptiveness, substance abuse, absenteeism, tardiness and so forth. These behaviours tend to cluster together (Sackett, 2002). Despite some differences in terminology, researchers agree that such behaviours are harmful to organisations and the people associated with them – in health services, these will be staff and patients.

Some recent research (Penney & Spector, 2002) investigates a previously unexplored link between narcissism and CWB. As we discussed earlier, narcissism has been defined as a form of high self-esteem, which is based on an inflated or grandiose self-image, sometimes linked to aggressive behaviour. Penney and Spector (2002) found that individuals high in narcissism reported feeling angry more often and reported engaging in more CWB than those lower in narcissism.

A problem in CWB research generally is the obvious difficulty in collecting accurate subjective data or objective observational data since much CWB is covert. This means that many of the correlations between CWB and narcissism, for example, may be underestimates. The types of CWB studied closely match the types of behaviours often found in poorly performing doctors, and indeed are cited as major sources of complaints (Sanger, 2000). A good indicator of the long-term nature of this behaviour comes in a study which considered all the graduates of a US medical school who had been disciplined by the local Medical Board over the previous decade, with controls matched by year and specialty choice (Papadakis *et al.*, 2004). Those disciplined were more likely to have had concerns raised about their behaviour, or actual unprofessional behaviour, recorded on their medical school file during their undergraduate years. This indicates a likelihood of such behaviours continuing, but also highlights the importance of good records passing from medical school to postgraduate training.

In conclusion, whilst it is difficult to generalise, it would appear that some underlying personality characteristics that may give rise to CWB are hard to alter. Interventions would almost certainly be time- and cost-intensive, and the behaviours unlikely to respond to short periods of coaching.

Insight and self-awareness

One of the most common complaints about doctors whose performance is giving cause for concern is their lack of insight into themselves and others.

A series of studies has shown that most of us overestimate our skills (Kruger & Dunning, 1999). People who are particularly *unskilled* in certain areas are actually *more* likely to overestimate their abilities. The authors see this as a deficit in the capacity to distinguish accuracy from error. They have shown that, although it sounds like a paradox, improving their skills actually increases their capacity to recognise their limitations better. This finding has been applied to medical students (Gruppen *et al.*, 2000), where the study showed that individual self-assessments were stable over time, regardless of performance. In other words, those who were poor at self-assessment stayed that way throughout the course (and perhaps longer) and vice versa.

However, there was an *overall fall* in accuracy (in both accurate and inaccurate students) when they began the more complex clinical work with patients, in which uncertainty continues to play a part throughout their careers. That is to say, where clinical work is concerned, most students are more likely to overestimate their skills. Whether this overestimation continues or not is an important research area, and it would also be useful to look at its relationship to self-criticism. Perhaps related to this finding is a study (Merrill *et al.*, 1994) which showed that those medical students with a low intolerance of ambiguity show over-reliance on technology, a negative view of psychological problems, and have a Machiavellian attitude that the 'means justify the end'. These students were more likely to favour surgery as a career.

This growing area of individual differences in self-awareness of skill levels and tolerance of uncertainty is likely to have implications for health professionals, particularly those working in some isolation where feedback may be less. In these days of error-reporting and learning from error, this may be particularly important to recognise, not only in terms of change and educational planning but also in the essential step of recognising that an error has been made at all. Nevertheless, the fact that accuracy of perception improves with increased skills is an encouraging finding.

Can psychological factors be changed or remedied?

There are indications from recent research in the occupational field which may provide useful guidance about the areas of personality and behaviour that may be more or less amenable to change. We see no reason why this guidance should not be applicable to doctors. Hogan and Warrenfeltz (2003) discuss individual differences in educability. From their work on executive learning they argue that three individual differences affect receptiveness:

1 **Self-control:** Those who are self-disciplined can focus, stay on task and concentrate on details (consistent with the Big Five research linking conscientiousness and training success (Barrick & Mount, 1991). Conversely, impulsive people are easily bored and distracted, have short attention spans, dislike details, and generally make poor students, unless they really care about the subject matter.
2 **Self-confidence:** This links with other work on grandiose self-esteem and low self-criticism (discussed earlier). It suggests that people with overinflated views

of their own ability may be less receptive to negative feedback. Paradoxically, those with low self-confidence who are highly self-critical are also hard to educate because they are alert for anything that sounds like criticism, and they become defensive when they hear it (Blatt & Zuroff, 1992). Because of their defensiveness, they have trouble testing their ideas about how others perceive them. Because they avoid negative feedback, they experience difficulty in reorganising their mental models. It is also argued that it is the people with average self-confidence who are the easiest to educate. They take reasonable responsibility and are willing to believe negative feedback, but they have enough self-confidence to try new ways of thinking and behaving. They will listen to criticism and feedback and use it well.

3 **Perceptiveness about others:** Those who understand what motivates others may be more receptive to learning. People differ quite substantially in terms of how insightful they are about other people (Hogan & Hogan, 2001). Linked to the studies of emotional intelligence (Goleman, 1998), perceptive people can quickly and intuitively understand what motivates others, and avoid management practices that gratuitously upset and alienate their staff. Research in this area is controversial. There is an increasing number of psychometric tools for identifying emotional intelligence with variable reliability and validity. Nevertheless, the concept is gaining currency in the management field as helpful in highlighting the impact of such attributes as empathy and sensitivity on managerial performance. These attributes are now accepted as part of the principles of the GMC's *Good Medical Practice*. More research is required to establish which measure of emotional intelligence could be useful in the medical context.

A number of psychological tests have done well in terms of predicting performance in some parts of medicine and in other settings. A fertile area for further research is to establish personality norms for doctors whose performance gives cause for concern, and compare these with norms developed for all doctors. This would help to identify more clearly the role of personality and attitudes in predicting a doctor's performance.

Conclusion

This review shows that there are potentially important ways that personality and other individual characteristics might be affecting performance and behaviour in medicine. In most areas these links are well established in other groups, but have rarely been applied within healthcare. Where they have been used in healthcare they follow the same pattern as elsewhere. Because of the rarity of this application, particularly within medicine, this review has not been able to be categorical about the implications for such areas as selection or adaptability. Nevertheless, the evidence from other areas is often strong and the implications for medicine are important. More than anything else, this review shows the need for a systematic research programme in this area.

References

Anastasi A and Urbin S (1997) *Psychological Testing*. Prentice-Hall, Englewood Cliffs, NJ.

Bardo MT, Donohew RL and Harrington NG (1996) Psychobiology of novelty seeking and drug seeking behaviour. *Behavioural Brain Research*. **77**(1–2): 23–43.

Barrick MR and Mount KM (1991) The Big Five personality dimensions and job performance: a meta-analysis. *Personnel Psychology*. **44**(1): 1–26.

Barrick MR, Mount KM and Judge TA (2001) Personality and performance at the beginning of the new millennium: what do we know and where do we go next? *International Journal of Selection and Assessment*. **9**(1–2): 9–30.

Bentz VJ (1985) *A View from the Top: a thirty year perspective of research devoted to the discovery, description and prediction of executive behaviour*. Paper presented at the 93rd Annual Convention of the American Psychological Association, Los Angeles, August.

Blatt SJ and Zuroff DC (1992) Interpersonal relatedness and self-definition: two proto-types for depression. *Clin Psychol Rev*. **12**: 527–62.

Brewin CR and Firth-Cozens J (1997) Dependency and self-criticism as predicting depression in young doctors. *Journal of Occupational Health Psychology*. **2**(3): 242–6.

Burns R and Sullivan P (2000) Perceptions of danger, risk taking, and outcomes in a remote community. *Environment and Behaviour*. **32**(1): 32–71.

Carthey J *et al.* (2003) Behavioural markers of surgical excellence. *Safety Science*. **41**(5): 409–25.

Clack GB *et al.* (2004) Personality differences between doctors and their patients: implications for the teaching of communications skills. *Medical Education*. **38**(2): 177–86.

Costa PT, McCrae RR and Zonderman AB (1987) Environmental and dispositional influences on well-being: longitudinal follow-up of an American national sample. *British Journal of Psychology*. **78**(3): 299–306.

DiMatteo MR *et al.* (1993) Physicians' characteristics influence patients' adherence to medical treatment – results from the Medical Outcomes study. *Health Psychology*. **12**(2): 93–102.

Firth-Cozens J (1985) Sources of stress in junior doctors and general practitioners. *Yorkshire Medicine*. **7**: 10–13.

Firth-Cozens J (1997) Depression in Doctors. In: C Katona and MM Robertson (eds) *Depression and Physical Illness*. Perspectives in Psychiatry Series. John Wiley & Sons, Chichester, pp. 95–111.

Firth-Cozens J and Cording H (2004) What matters more in patient care? Giving doctors shorter hours of work or a good night's sleep? *Quality & Safety in Health Care*. **13**(3): 165–6.

Firth-Cozens J, Lema VC and Firth RA (1999) Specialty choice, stress and personality: their relationships over time. *Hospital Medicine*. **60**(10): 751–5.

Firth-Cozens J and Mowbray D (2001) Leadership and the quality of care. *Quality in Health Care*. **10**(Suppl 2): 3–7.

Flett GL and Hewitt PL (eds) (2002) *Perfectionism: theory, research and treatment*. American Psychological Association, Washington, DC.

Gibbons RD, Gudas C and Gibbons SW (1983) A study of the relationship between flexibility of closure and surgical skill. *Journal of the American Podiatry Association*. **73**(1): 12–16.

Goleman D (1998) *Working with Emotional Intelligence*. Bloomsbury, New York.

Gough HG, Bradley P and McDonald JS (1991) Performance of residents in anesthesiology as related to measures of personality and interests. *Psychological Reports*. **68**(3 part 1): 979–94.

Greene K *et al.* (2000) Targeting adolescent risk-taking behaviors: the contributions of egocentrism and sensation-seeking. *Journal of Adolescence*. **23**(4): 439–61.

Gruppen LD *et al.* (2000) Medical students' self-assessments and their allocations of learning time. *Academic Medicine*. **75**(4): 374–9.

Hall JC, Ellis C and Hamdorf J (2003) Surgeons and cognitive processes. *British Journal of Surgery.* **90**(1): 10–16.

Helmreich RL *et al.* (1986) Cockpit resource management: exploring the attitude-performance linkage. *Aviation, Space, and Environmental Medicine.* **57**(12): 1198–200.

Helmreich RL and Wilhelm JA (1991) Outcomes of crew resource management training. *International Journal of Aviation Psychology.* **1**(4): 287–300.

Hogan R and Hogan J (1997) *Hogan Development Survey Manual.* Hogan Assessment Systems, Tulsa, OK.

Hogan R and Hogan J (2001) Assessing leadership: a view from the dark side. *International Journal of Selection and Assessment.* **9**(1–2): 40–51.

Hogan R and Warrenfeltz R (2003) Educating the Modern Manager. *Academy of Management Learning and Education.* **2**(1): 2–30.

Horney K (1950) *Neurosis and Human Growth.* Norton, New York.

Horvath P and Zuckerman M (1993) Sensation seeking, risk appraisal and risky behaviour. *Personality and Individual Differences.* **14**(1): 41–52.

Hoyle RH (2000) Personality processes and problem behavior. *Journal of Personality.* **68**(6): 953–66.

Hunter JE and Hunter RF (1984) Validity and utility of alternative predictors of job performance. *Psychological Bulletin.* **96**(1): 72–98.

Kroeger O and Thuesen JM (1989) *Type Talk: the 16 personality types that determine how we live, love and work.* Dell, New York.

Kruger J and Dunning D (1999) Unskilled and unaware of it: how difficulties in recognizing one's own incompetence lead to inflated self-assessments. *Journal of Personality and Social Psychology.* **77**(6): 1121–34.

Leslie JB and Van Velsor EA (1997) *A Look at Derailment Today: North America and Europe.* Center for Creative Leadership, Greensboro, NC.

Linn BS and Zeppa R (1982) Values and attitudes related to career preference and performance in the surgical clerkship. *Archives of Surgery.* **117**(10): 1276–80.

Linn LS *et al.* (1985) Physician and patient satisfaction as factors related to the organization of internal medicine group practices. *Medical Care.* **23**(10): 1171–8.

McCall MW and Lombardo MM (1983) *Off The Track: why and how successful executives get derailed.* Center for Creative Leadership, Greensboro, NC.

McDonald J, Orlick T and Letts M (1995) Mental readiness in surgeons and its links to performance excellence in surgery. *Journal of Pediatric Orthopedics.* **15**(5): 691–7.

Merrill JM *et al.* (1994) Uncertainties and ambiguities: measuring how medical students cope. *Medical Education.* **28**(4): 316–22.

Millon T and Davis R (2000) *Personality Disorders in Modern Life.* John Wiley & Sons, New York.

Norris FH, Smith T and Kaniasty K (1999) Revisiting the experience-behavior hypothesis: the effect of Hurricane Hugo on hazard preparedness and other self-protective acts. *Basic and Applied Social Psychology.* **21**(1): 37–47.

O'Connor RC and O'Connor DB (2003) Predicting hopelessness and psychological distress: the role of perfectionism and coping. *Journal of Counseling Psychology.* **50**(3): 362–72.

Ones DS, Viswesvaran C and Schmidt FL (1993) Comprehensive meta-analysis of integrity test validities: findings and implications for personnel selection and theories of job performance. *Journal of Applied Psychology.* **78**(4): 679–703.

Ostroff C (1992) The relationship between satisfaction, attitudes, and performance: an organizational level analysis. *Journal of Applied Psychology.* **77**(6): 963–74.

Paice E and Firth-Cozens J (2003) Who's a bully then? *BMJ.* **326**(7393): S127.

Papadakis MA *et al.* (2004) Unprofessional behavior in medical school is associated with subsequent disciplinary action by a state medical board. *Academic Medicine.* **79**(3): 244–9.

Papps BP and O'Carroll RE (1998) Extremes of self-esteem and narcissism and the experience and expression of anger and aggression. *Aggressive Behavior.* **24**(6): 421–38.

Penney LM and Spector PE (2002) Narcissism and counterproductive work behavior: do bigger egos mean bigger problems? *International Journal of Selection and Assessment.* **10**(1–2): 126–34.

Perry AR and Baldwin DA (2000) Further evidence of associations of type A personality scores and driving related attitudes and behaviors. *Perceptual and Motor Skills.* **91**(1): 147–54.

Pinkerton SD and Abramson PR (1995) Decision-making and personality factors in sexual risk-taking for HIV/AIDS: a theoretical integration. *Personality and Individual Differences.* **19**(5): 713–23.

Rabaud C *et al.* (2000) Occupational exposure to blood: search for a relation between personality and behaviour. *Infection Control and Hospital Epidemiology.* **21**(9): 564–74.

Reeve PE, Vickers MD and Horton JN (1993) Selecting anaesthetists: the use of psychological tests and structured interviews. *Journal of the Royal Society of Medicine.* **86**(7): 400–5.

Rochlin GI (1999) Safe operation as a social construct. *Ergonomics.* **42**(11): 1549–60.

Sackett PR (2002) The structure of counterproductive work behaviours: dimensionality and relationships with facets of job performance. *International Journal of Selection & Assessment.* **10**(1–2): 5–11.

Salmivalli C (2001) Feeling good about oneself, being bad to others? Remarks on self-esteem, hostility and aggressive behaviour. *Aggression and Violent Behavior.* **6**(4): 375–93.

Sanger J (2000) Putting the person in appraisal. *Clinician in Management.* **9**(4): 195.

Schaper M (2002) Small firms and environmental management: predictors of green purchasing in Western Australian pharmacies. *International Small Business Journal.* **20**(3): 235–51.

Schneider B and Bowen DE (1985) Employee and customer perceptions of service in banks: replication and extension. *Journal of Applied Psychology.* **70**(3): 423–33.

Sexton JB, Thomas EJ and Helmreich RL (2000) Error, stress and teamwork in medicine and aviation: cross sectional surveys. *BMJ.* **320**(7237): 745–9.

Sicard B, Jouve E and Blin O (2001) Risk propensity assessment in military specials operations. *Military Medicine.* **166**(10): 871–4.

Slovic P (1987) Perception of risk. *Science.* **236**: 280–5.

Smith SL and Friedland DS (1998) The influence of education and personality on risk propensity in nurse managers. *Journal of Nursing Administration.* **28**(12): 22–7.

Stevenson H and Henley S (1989) *Job Analysis Report on the Role of the Surgeon.* Saville and Holdsworth Ltd, Thames Ditton.

Stewart WH and Roth PL (2001) Risk propensity differences between entrepreneurs and managers: a meta-analytic review. *Journal of Applied Psychology.* **86**(1): 145–53.

Waldron I *et al.* (1980) Type A behavior pattern: relationship to variation in blood pressure, parental characteristics and academic and social activities of students. *Journal of Human Stress.* **6**(1): 16–27.

Zuckerman M and Kuhlman M (2000) Personality and risk-taking: common biosocial factors. *Journal of Personality.* **68**(6): 999–1029.

Chapter 6

The role of education and training

Elisabeth Paice

Introduction

This chapter reviews the evidence that educational factors, before and after quali-fication, have an impact on the performance of doctors. Do the attributes of students entering medical school predict their subsequent performance? Does the curriculum or teaching style favoured by the school make any difference? What are the features of an effective postgraduate training programme, and what are the obstacles to learning? Can poor performance be prevented, predicted, detected early or remediated within the undergraduate, postgraduate and continuing pro-fessional development system in place in the UK?

The factors within education, training, appraisal and continuing professional development (CPD) are summarised in Figure 6.1.

Basic medical education

Attributes of medical school entrants and their subsequent performance

Most medical schools would wish to turn away any applicants who were unlikely to turn into caring, conscientious and competent doctors. The challenge is to know how to recognise them. Admission to medical school is competitive in most countries, and most of those applying have good scholastic records and are scien-tifically inclined. Selecting from this pool is difficult and a great deal of research has gone into looking at the factors that predict success in completing the course. Less is known about the factors that predict subsequent clinical performance. The UK Committee of Deans and Heads of Medical Schools commissioned a systematic review of factors believed to be significant predictors of success in medicine. The review examined data on the predictive validity of eight criteria that have been studied in relation to the selection of medical students: cognitive factors (previous academic ability), non-cognitive factors (personality, learning styles, interviews, references, personal statements) and demographic factors (sex, ethnicity). They found that previous academic performance was a good, but not perfect, predictor of achievement in medical training, accounting for 23% of the variance in perform-ance in undergraduate medical training and 6% of the variance in postgraduate competency. A strategic learning style, white ethnicity and female sex were all also associated with success in medical training (Ferguson, James & Madeley, 2002). Having said that, a rich and complex social, ethnic and class mix results in more socially able graduates (McManus, 2003; Crosby *et al.*, 2003).

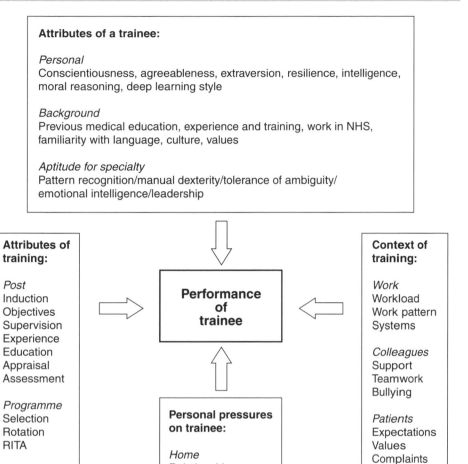

Attributes of a trainee:

Personal
Conscientiousness, agreeableness, extraversion, resilience, intelligence, moral reasoning, deep learning style

Background
Previous medical education, experience and training, work in NHS, familiarity with language, culture, values

Aptitude for specialty
Pattern recognition/manual dexterity/tolerance of ambiguity/ emotional intelligence/leadership

Attributes of training:

Post
Induction
Objectives
Supervision
Experience
Education
Appraisal
Assessment

Programme
Selection
Rotation
RITA

Performance of trainee

Context of training:

Work
Workload
Work pattern
Systems

Colleagues
Support
Teamwork
Bullying

Patients
Expectations
Values
Complaints

Personal pressures on trainee:

Home
Relationships
Childcare
Elderly parents
Financial concerns

Health
Substance abuse
Mental illness
Physical illness
Disability

Figure 6.1 Factors impacting on the performance of trainees.

Predicting clinical performance after graduation is more difficult. Selection of medical students has tended to depend heavily on A-level or similar exam results, because intelligence and conscientiousness are needed for success during medical school, and exam results assess a combination of these two important but unrelated factors. Subsequent postgraduate performance requires enough intellectual ability to do the job, conscientiousness and integrity. Helpfulness and willingness to co-operate come close behind, along with interpersonal skills and empathy. Psychological stability and resilience are also important in a profession vulnerable to alcoholism, drug abuse and suicide (Hughes, 2002).

Although some scholastic tests such as the Medical Colleges Admission Test in the USA do not predict clinical performance (Reede, 1999), a UK 20-year longitudinal study found that A-level scores were a predictor for medical career success. Although the results of an intelligence test did not correlate with career success, A-levels did, possibly because of the knowledge acquired, the conscientiousness required or because A-levels are designed to reward deep learning styles, rather than learning by rote (McManus *et al.*, 2003). Deep learning, when a student's imagination is captured and he or she pursues knowledge for its intrinsic interest, is not encouraged by high-stakes assessments.

Other studies have shown a relationship between personality type and sub-sequent medical career success, with agreeable, stable extroverted types perform-ing better and enjoying their careers more than neurotic introverts. Resilience in the face of stress is an important attribute for doctors. Students with elevated stress and depression often seek out particular careers, but may continue to suffer from stress. For example, those who were stressed as students appear to favour psychiatry or laboratory medicine. Doctors who chose laboratory medicine stay depressed but become less stressed, whilst those in psychiatry remain the most stressed and depressed (Firth-Cozens, Lema & Firth, 1999).

Psychometric testing has been advocated to select the ideal personality for a medical career, but since these tests depend on self-reporting, they are not reliable instruments for selection once the word gets out about the personality types being selected for admission to medical school. Other instruments are constantly being developed. In one promising study, scores on a written moral reasoning test were shown to correlate with performance, and were inversely related to malpractice claims among orthopaedic surgeons (Self & Baldwin, 2000). As longitudinal studies reveal more and more evidence about the attributes of medical school applicants that predict subsequent clinical performance, medical school admissions pro-cedures must adjust to reflect these. However, the impact of such changes in the selection of students on the subsequent performance of practising doctors will inevitably be slow.

Learning styles and performance

Some students perform well and others struggle to pass their assessments and exams. Assessments in medical school tend to carry high stakes, and raise anxieties about failure. Under these circumstances superficial rote learning (e.g. memorising lists) is, for some students, inevitable, as is strategic learning (e.g. preparing for likely questions). However, it is deep learning that is most likely to lead to retention of knowledge, and that forms the best basis for lifelong learning once the stimulus of examinations is over. There is some evidence that less able students have a surface rather than deep learning style and are motivated by fear of failure rather than a desire to master the subject (McManus, Richards & Winder, 1999). On graduation, surface learners are more likely to have negative attitudes to work and continuing education. They tend to feel overworked, unsupported and prevented from taking up educational opportunities by numerous obstacles (Delva *et al.*, 2002). Learning styles tend to be stable, but can change. For example, doing an intercalated BSc caused a proportion of surface learners to adopt a deeper learning style which was subsequently maintained (McManus, Keeling & Paice, 2004).

The curriculum

Medical school should prepare a doctor for a lifetime of practice and continued learning. Although the knowledge, skills and attitudes learned in medical school will date, a commitment to keep abreast of important developments, to hone skills and to accept that other skills will grow too rusty to use, and to keep in touch with the values of society will help doctors to maintain good medical practice throughout their careers.

Medical schools in the UK approach their tasks in different ways, but the General Medical Council (GMC) ensures consistency in the curriculum, and the examining bodies ensure that standards are maintained. While changes in the curriculum may impact on the students' sense of readiness for clinical practice on graduation (Jones, McArdle & O'Neill, 2002), there is no evidence that any one UK medical school is more likely to produce poorly performing doctors than another. There is, however, recent evidence that the graduates of some US medical schools are consistently more likely to be the subject of malpractice claims than others (Waters, Lefevre & Budetti, 2003). Whether this reflects the admissions policy, the relative popularity, or the quality of the learning environment of the medical schools is not known, although the outlying schools were more likely to be new and publicly funded.

Topics such as communications skills were rarely taught before the GMC published *Tomorrow's Doctors* (General Medical Council, 2003), but are now part of the standard curriculum. Communications training improves students' overall communications competence as well as their skills in relationship building, organisation and time management, patient assessment, negotiation and shared decision-making tasks that are important to positive patient outcomes (Yedidia *et al.*, 2003). Professional values and attitudes are also part of the curriculum defined by *Tomorrow's Doctors* (General Medical Council, 2003) and of the GMC's guidance for all doctors, *Good Medical Practice* (General Medical Council, 2001). Values have to be adjusted as society changes. For example, respect for diversity is now accepted as an important professional value, but only recently have graduates covered this as part of their curriculum at medical school. Doctors who graduated in the sixties or seventies, or graduates from medical schools in other countries, may well have had attitudes instilled in them that sit uneasily with current medical practice in the UK. A paternalistic approach to patient care, an expectation that it is the doctor who should always lead other healthcare workers, and a refusal to take resources into account when dealing with an individual patient are examples of attitudes that may lead a conscientious and committed doctor into trouble in today's health service.

Teaching professional values

Although the teaching of professional values and medical ethics is a compulsory component of the new curriculum, the teaching may be undermined by what students observe in practice (Feudtner, Christakis & Christakis, 1994). Some physicians refer to patients in a derogatory manner, or behave in a way that is ethically reprehensible (Paice *et al.*, 2002a). These doctors are unlikely to be clinically excellent and do not make safe role models for students or trainees (Rhoton, 1994). Not all experienced doctors can be depended upon to teach professional values, attitudes and behaviours by example (Paice, Heard & Moss, 2002). Doctors who behave unethically should not be entrusted with trainees.

Assessment and examinations

The final examination is the point at which students prove their readiness to become doctors. Scores achieved on certification and licensure examinations taken at the end of medical school show a sustained relationship, over 4 to 7 years, with indices of preventive care and acute and chronic disease management in primary care practice (Tamblyn *et al.*, 2002). However, traditional final examinations are not as good as Objective Structured Clinical Examinations (OSCEs) in predicting the performance of recent graduates in their pre-registration house officer year (Probert *et al.*, 2003). A move to more OSCE-based examinations is occurring and should be welcomed.

Fitness to practise and transfer of information

Traditionally medical students have been allowed more latitude in their behaviour than would be acceptable in registered practitioners. Youthful high spirits, including drunkenness and anti-social behaviour, have been tolerated. Recently, however, and as a result of some extreme examples of irresponsibility, procedures have been put into place to review medical students and pre-registration house officers whose behaviour or health calls into question their fitness to practise. Despite passing their qualifying examinations, in extreme cases such individuals are not allowed to become fully registered medical practitioners. In less extreme cases, information about a new graduate is transferred from medical school to those supervising their first Pre-Registration House Officer (PRHO) or intern post. The purpose of such information is to identify students who are at risk of becoming poor performers and who may need extra support. A transfer of information system has been developed and implemented successfully by Imperial College London. Students complete a form summarising their medical school career in terms of exams, performance, health and behaviour, which is sent to the clinical tutor of the hospital where they are to work. The results of the first two years suggest that students do not falsify their reports and that useful information is transferred by this route, although students have expressed concern about having to provide negative information about themselves (Frankel & English, 2004).

The pre-registration year

A tough transition

The first experience of working as a doctor can come as a shock. Final-year students are responsible only for themselves. They decide when to go to sleep and when to get up, when to study and when to relax. They are at the top of the medical student hierarchy. As new house officers, they are at the bottom of the medical hierarchy. There are jobs that must be done and the needs of patients come before the most basic and pressing of personal needs. Virtually everyone seems to be authorised to order them about. On top of that, they have to cope with being very close to the human tragedies of disease and death, often with little time, support or recognition of their understandable distress (Paice *et al.*, 2002b). Pressures in the organisation often prevent new doctors from having control over their work or time for reflection.

The consequence may be disillusionment and depression, especially for those young doctors with high empathy and self-criticism. Any improvements in organisations' approach to quality improvement must recognise the tendency of healthcare professionals to respond to stress by increasing personal detachment, even to the point of dehumanising patients. This coping strategy is learned early and unlearned with difficulty (Firth-Cozens, 1992). Inevitably some new doctors fail to cope with this transition and stress levels in the PRHO year are high, with up to 30% demonstrating evidence of psychological morbidity. When this happens, it is rarely lack of factual knowledge that lets them down but a lack of preparedness for the discipline of the world of work.

The concept of the poorly performing PRHO is a relatively new one. Until recently the GMC only required to know that the compulsory experiential elements of the year had been completed, not how well. It was rare for a PRHO to be required to repeat any element of the year before being signed up, other than because of sick leave. This has changed and 1–2% of PRHOs are now required to undertake remedial training before being signed up. It is likely that this is the result of closer supervision and scrutiny, rather than a sharp deterioration in the performance of PRHOs.

PRHOs are the source of a disproportionate share of drug errors in hospital, and contribute to the worrying morbidity and mortality from this cause. To reduce prescribing errors, hospitals should prepare, train and supervise junior doctors in the principles of prescribing, and enforce good practice in documentation. They should also create a culture in which prescription writing is seen as important as well as formally reviewing locum arrangements, interventions made by pharmacists and the workload of junior doctors. They should make doctors aware of situations in which they are likely to commit errors (Dean *et al.*, 2002).

Postgraduate education and training

The educational framework

Postgraduate training used to be a matter of experience gained under supervision while preparing for external examinations. Progress from grade to grade was dependent on patronage and it was expected that a proportion of trainees would fail to make the cut at each level. No special arrangements were in place to deal with these failures, although Lord Moran famously and offensively suggested that general practice consisted of those who had fallen off the specialist ladder. Things have changed. Over the past two decades, reforms of postgraduate training have been introduced to make the selection process more transparent, consistent and fair (Heard *et al.*, 2002). Entry criteria to each specialty have been defined, a curriculum published, and an assessment process developed (Department of Health, 1993). These changes have mainly concerned the registrar (GP or specialist) grade, but have also affected the senior house officer grade (Paice & Leaver, 1999). Under the title *Modernising Medical Careers* the UK government is changing the structure of postgraduate medical education. The educational framework (Box 6.1) which has underpinned the reforms of specialist training (Paice *et al.*, 2000; Paice & Ginsburg, 2003) will be implemented for all trainees, whatever their grade.

Appraisal

All learners need feedback on their progress, and doctors in training express more satisfaction with their training if they have the opportunity to sit down with a supervising consultant and talk about how they are doing. The majority of trainees report that such discussions are useful, especially if they are based on observed performance, a log book or some other objective evidence (Paice *et al.*, 1997; Paice & Aitken, 2004). Appraisal is intended to be a supportive, developmental, two-way discussion of progress, resulting in objectives for the next phase of training. Training in appraisal skills is provided for educational supervisors, by deaneries, by employers and on-line.

Box 6.1 The educational framework

1 **Induction:** to the organisation (e.g. hospital) and to the immediate working environment (e.g. department) for each placement.
2 **Objectives setting:** agreeing which elements of the curriculum are to be mastered within this placement. Documented in a **training (or learning) agreement** in which the objectives and how they are to be achieved are set down, and the responsibilities of both trainer and trainee are made explicit.
3 **Supervision:** learning while doing under the eye of a senior who is competent both to do the task and to train others.
4 **Experience:** the opportunity to learn while doing a range of appropriate procedures, or caring for patients with a variety of conditions, tailored to the level of competence achieved. Documented in a **log book** – a record kept by trainees and discussed with their supervisor of procedures done, competencies achieved, etc.
5 **Education:** regular, timetabled sessions at which topics relevant to the trainee are discussed away from the clinical setting.
6 **Appraisal:** a regular, planned meeting with an educational supervisor at which informed feedback is given to the trainee about their performance against the agreed objectives, obstacles are discussed, problems aired and new objectives set.
7 **Assessment:** an objective evaluation of the trainee's knowledge, skills and/or behaviour, based on observed performance in the workplace or on the results of a test or series of tests. A record of the in-training assessments acquired by a Specialist Registrar (SpR) in the course of a year is reviewed by a panel and a summary evaluation is made as to whether these represent sufficient evidence of satisfactory progress to allow progress to the next stage of training, or whether targeted or repeat training is required.

Assessment

Assessment of clinical knowledge, skills, attitudes, competence and performance is not easy. Some principles emerge from the literature on the subject. No one assessment method is robust on its own and a large sample of items are needed to obtain adequate reliability. A robust assessment will include objective testing of a range of domains (e.g. clinical, technical, interpersonal, organisational, ethical etc.), using a range of methods or instruments (e.g. observed practice, notes review, OSCE or Multiple Choice Question (MCQ) test) by a range of assessors (e.g. consultants, peers, colleagues). The assessments should be related to the curriculum for the specialty, and ideally the Royal College concerned should provide help with descriptors of standards to be attained at various stages, and appropriate instruments to be used (Wragg *et al.*, 2003; Martin *et al.*, 1997).

There are substantial gaps in the definition and assessment of professional performance, particularly systems management and personal development. These include: how well individuals collaborate with other health professionals to achieve desired outcomes (teamwork); how well patients of individual doctors improve their knowledge and understanding of their health (empowerment); how individuals keep up-to-date with new developments (maintaining currency of practice); and the degree to which individual doctors are aware of their strengths and weaknesses (insight) (Newble *et al.*, 1994).

Early signs of the trainee in difficulty

Managing the trainee whose performance is causing concern is a difficult task, especially if the trainee demonstrates lack of insight or recognition that there are problems. Early warning signs of problems may be soft and difficult to articulate. During a series of workshops on trainees in difficulty, certain features were repeatedly identified as the first indication of problems in trainees who subsequently ran into serious difficulty (*see* Box 6.2). Any of these signs should trigger a heightened level of supervision, and attention to the possibility of ill health, psychological distress, substance abuse or other factors that may be responsible for this behaviour.

Box 6.2 Early signs of trainees in difficulty

- **The disappearing act:** not answering bleeps; disappearing between clinic and ward; lateness; excessive amounts of sick leave.
- **Low workrate:** slowness at procedures, clerkings, dictating letters, making decisions; coming early and staying late and still not getting a reasonable workload done.
- **Ward rage:** bursts of temper when decisions questioned; shouting matches with colleagues or patients; real or imagined slights.
- **Rigidity:** poor tolerance of ambiguity; inability to compromise; difficulty prioritising; inappropriate 'whistle-blowing'.
- **Bypass syndrome:** junior colleagues or nurses finding ways to avoid seeking their opinion or help.
- **Career problems:** difficulty with exams; uncertainty about career choice; disillusionment with medicine.
- **Insight failure:** rejection of constructive criticism; defensiveness; counter-challenge.

Poor performance and assessment in postgraduate training

The introduction of systematic assessment during postgraduate training (the Record of In Training Assessment (RITA) process) in 1995 was intended to ensure that every specialist registrar had an annual assessment of their progress, followed by a documented recommendation that they were ready to progress to the next year of a structured programme, needed targeted training, or needed to repeat training at the same level. Repeated failure to progress would lead to withdrawal from the programme. Successful completion of the full programme would lead to a recommendation to the Specialist Training Authority that a Certificate of Completion of Specialist Training (CCST) be issued (NHS Executive, 1995). This process is currently being extended to other grades, despite concerns that there are problems as yet unresolved with its application to the SpR grade (Paice, 1999).

Individuals learn and mature at different rates, and inevitably some trainees will not achieve the required standard of competence within a timeframe defined as the minimum required. Whether slow developers should be considered to be poor performers is questionable. Depending on their insight, trainees who are identified as needing more time, and offered repeat training, are either grateful or resentful. It would be easier for such trainees to accept the verdict if there was no stigma attached, but delay is seen as failure and is often passionately contested. Sometimes the outcome has been withdrawal from the training programme, voluntary or enforced (Tunbridge, Dickinson & Swan, 2002). Under these circumstances, it is small wonder that the RITA process is perceived as a high-stakes assessment which may impinge on the trainee's human right to work. Under such circumstances the standard of proof required is high, and the assessment systems in place are rarely 'appeal-proof', especially when counter-claims are made of flawed educational frameworks, inadequate workplace assessments, racial or sexual discrimination or workplace bullying. When repeat and remedial training fail, questions arise as to the suitability of the trainee for an alternative career in another branch of medicine or whether they are suited to being doctors at all.

Insight and poor performance

While there is little evidence to suggest that the majority of doctors do not maintain a reasonable level of performance in current practice, more is known about those doctors investigated after reports of poor practice. Common findings in the assessment of such doctors include professional isolation, lack of awareness of their poor performance and substantial gaps in their knowledge and skills. Such doctors prove to be difficult to remediate and may leave medical practice. This raises the question as to whether all doctors with performance problems should be assessed for insight in order to determine their capacity for remediation. The differences between self- and external assessments might represent an important measure of capacity to change, inferring a kind of insight or change 'gap' (Hays *et al.*, 2002).

Against that proposal is fascinating evidence that people who perform least well in tests of competence tend to rate their performance as above average, while the best performers rate themselves only a little more highly (Kruger & Dunning, 1999). The explanation appears to be that poor performers have less insight into the inadequacy of their own performance, while top performers have excessive expectations of the performance of their peers. This finding helps to explain the gulf in understanding that sometimes opens up between a highly competent team member and a less talented colleague. Even more interesting is the finding that, when training is given to poor performers, they revise their self-rating downward, despite performing better. In other words, the more training they are offered, and the more competent they become, the more insight they develop into their shortcomings. This research is a powerful argument against using lack of insight as a reason for dismissing the possibility of successful remedial training.

Bullying and performance

There has been a recent rise in awareness of workplace bullying as a cause of poor performance. Medicine has always been a hierarchical environment and senior doctors have had their juniors' careers in their gift. With such an imbalance of power, abuses were inevitable. This situation is changing, but bullying of trainees by their consultants remains a common feature of hospital life (Hicks, 2000; Quine, 2002). A recent survey showed that 18% of trainees had experienced persistent behaviour by others that undermined their self-confidence and professional self-esteem, within their current post. The more junior the respondent, the more likely they were to have experienced this, and the more likely the perpetrator was to be a more senior trainee (Paice, Houghton & Firth-Cozens, in preparation). It is likely that much of the behaviour experienced as bullying is intended to improve performance, not to erode confidence. An educational rather than punitive approach is needed to alter the behaviour of those who may be an unwitting source of distress to junior colleagues (Paice & Firth-Cozens, 2003).

Training and employment

Virtually all postgraduate training in the UK takes place within the context of paid employment, often in a series of posts with more than one employer, but under the management of, and funded by, the postgraduate deanery. There is inevitably a blurring of boundaries between employment and training, especially when a doctor in training performs poorly. Questions arise as to whether the problem should be dealt with as a training or disciplinary matter. Trusts are increasingly reluctant to embark on disciplinary procedures, which are often prolonged and costly (Goldman & Lewis, 2003). They may prefer the deanery to remove the trainee and place him or her elsewhere, rather than going through the process of investigating complaints. While this is understandable, it is unsatisfactory, especially for the trainee who has not had the opportunity to defend him- or herself (Paice, Orton & Appleyard, 1999).

Continuing professional development

Lifelong learning is an inevitable requirement for practice in a profession where advances are accelerating and societal attitudes are undergoing a revolution. Continuing professional development needs to be relevant to the context in which the doctor works. To as great an extent as possible, it should be evidence-based. For effective learning to proceed, achievement of the desired outcome must be perceived either as realistic or as divisible into manageable learning steps, and as transformable into a learning plan (Handfield-Jones *et al.*, 2002). Where perform-ance has slipped beyond a certain point the effort required to regain an acceptable level may be just too daunting to be contemplated (Bahrami & Evans, 2001). It remains to be seen whether assessment of competence, as part of the process of revalidation and relicensure in the UK, is regarded by practising doctors as high-stakes and threatening, or as helpful in focusing attention on their areas of need.

References

Bahrami J and Evans A (2001) Underperforming doctors in general practice: a survey of referrals to UK Deaneries. *British Journal of General Practice.* **51**(472): 892–6.

Crosby FJ *et al.* (2003) Affirmative action: psychological data and the policy debates. *American Psychologist.* **58**(2): 93–115.

Dean B *et al.* (2002) Causes of prescribing errors in hospital inpatients: a prospective study. *The Lancet.* **359**(9315): 1373–8.

Delva MD *et al.* (2002) Postal survey of approaches to learning among Ontario physicians: implications for continuing medical education. *BMJ.* **325**(7374): 1218.

Department of Health (1993) *Hospital Doctors: training for the future.* Department of Health, London.

Ferguson E, James D and Madeley L (2002) Factors associated with success in medical school: systematic review of the literature. *BMJ.* **324**(7343): 952–7.

Feudtner C, Christakis DA and Christakis NA (1994) Do clinical clerks suffer ethical erosion? Students' perceptions of their ethical environment and personal development. *Academic Medicine.* **69**(8): 670–9.

Firth-Cozens J (1992) The role of early family experiences in the perception of organizational stress: fusing clinical and organizational perspectives. *Journal of Occupational and Organizational Psychology.* **65**(1): 61–75.

Firth-Cozens J, Lema VC and Firth RA (1999) Specialty choice, stress and personality: their relationships over time. *Hospital Medicine.* **60**(10): 751–5.

Frankel A and English S (2004) Transfer of information from medical schools. *Hospital Medicine.* **65**(3): 170–3.

General Medical Council (2001) *Good Medical Practice* [online] (3e). www.gmc-uk.org/standards/default.htm [Accessed on 22 September 2004].

General Medical Council (2003) *Tomorrow's Doctors: recommendations on undergraduate medical education* [online]. General Medical Council. www.gmcuk.org/med_ed/tomdoc.htm [Accessed 22 September 2004].

Goldman L and Lewis J (2003) Cases of professional and personal conduct. *Employing Doctors and Dentists.* **July/August:** 5.

Handfield-Jones RS *et al.* (2002) Linking assessment to learning: a new route to quality assurance in medical practice. *Medical Education.* **36**(10): 949–58.

Hays BC *et al.* (2002) Is insight important? Measuring capacity to change performance. *Medical Education.* **36**(10): 965–71.

Heard S *et al.* (2002) Using a competence framework to select future medical specialists. *Hospital Medicine.* **63**(6): 361–7.

Hicks B (2000) Time to stop bullying and intimidation. *Hospital Medicine.* **61**(6): 428–31.

Hughes P (2002) Can we improve on how we select medical students? *Journal of the Royal Society of Medicine.* **95**(1): 18–22.

Jones A, McArdle PJ and O'Neill PA (2002) Perceptions of how well graduates are prepared for the role of pre-registration house officer: a comparison of outcomes from a traditional and an integrated PBL curriculum. *Medical Education.* **36**(1): 16–25.

Kruger J and Dunning D (1999) Unskilled and unaware of it: how difficulties in recognising one's own incompetence lead to inflated self-assessments. *Journal of Personality and Social Psychology.* **77**(6): 1121–34.

Martin JA *et al.* (1997) Objective structured assessment of technical skill (OSATS) for surgical residents. *British Journal of Surgery.* **84**(2): 273–8.

McManus IC (2003) Medical school differences: beneficial diversity or harmful deviations? *Quality & Safety in Health Care.* **12**(5): 324–5.

McManus IC *et al.* (2003) A levels and intelligence as predictors of medical careers in UK doctors: 20 year prospective study. *BMJ.* **327**(7407): 139–42.

McManus IC, Richards P and Winder BC (1999) Intercalated degrees, learning styles and career preferences: prospective longitudinal study of UK medical students. *BMJ.* **319**(7209): 542–6.

McManus IC, Keeling A and Paice E (2004) Stress, burnout and doctors' attitudes to work are determined by personality and learning style: a twelve year longitudinal study of UK medical graduates. *BMC Medicine [electronic resource].* **2**(1): 29.

Newble D *et al.* (1994) Guidelines for the development of effective and efficient procedures for the assessment of clinical competence. In: D Newble, B Jolly and R Wakeford (eds) *The Certification and Recertification of Doctors: issues in the assessment of clinical competence.* Cambridge University Press, Cambridge, pp. 69–91.

NHS Executive (1995) *A Guide to Specialist Registrar Training.* NHS Executive, Leeds.

Paice E (1999) *RITA – have we got it right?* Paper for STA.

Paice E *et al.* (1997) Association of use of a log book and experience as a pre-registration house officer: interview survey. *BMJ.* **314**(7075): 213–15.

Paice E *et al.* (2000) Trainee satisfaction before and after the Calman reforms of specialist training: questionnaire survey. *BMJ.* **320**(7238): 832–6.

Paice E *et al.* (2002a) The relationship between pre-registration house officers and their consultants. *Medical Education.* **36**(1): 26–34.

Paice E *et al.* (2002b) Stressful incidents, stress and coping strategies in the pre-registration house officer year. *Medical Education.* **36**(1): 56–65.

Paice E and Aitken M (2004) *South London Trainees' Point Of View Survey 2003/2004* [online]. London Department of Postgraduate Medical & Dental Education. www.londondeanery.ac.uk/publications/PointOfViewSurvey/index.asp [Accessed on 22 September 2004].

Paice E and Firth-Cozens J (2003) Who's a bully then? *BMJ.* **326**(7393): S127.

Paice E and Ginsburg R (2003) Specialist registrar training: what still needs to be improved? *Hospital Medicine.* **64**(3): 173–6.

Paice E, Heard SR and Moss F (2002) How important are role models in making good doctors? *BMJ.* **325**(7366): 707–10.

Paice E, Houghton A and Firth-Cozens J. Bullying amongst doctors in training: the pecking order at work. In preparation.

Paice E and Leaver P (1999) Improving the training of SHOs. *BMJ.* **318**(7190): 1022–3.

Paice E, Orton V and Appleyard J (1999) Managing trainee doctors in difficulty. *Hospital Medicine.* **60**(2): 130–3.

Probert CS *et al.* (2003) Traditional finals and OSCEs in predicting consultant and self-reported clinical skills of PRHOs: a pilot study. *Medical Education.* **37**(7): 597–602.

Quine L (2002) Workplace bullying in junior doctors: questionnaire survey. *BMJ.* **324**(7342): 878–9.

Reede JY (1999) Predictors of success in medicine. *Clinical Orthopaedics and Related Research.* **362**: 72–7.

Rhoton MF (1994) Professionalism and clinical excellence among anesthesiology residents. *Academic Medicine.* **69**(4): 313–15.

Self DJ and Baldwin DC Jr (2000) Should moral reasoning serve as a criterion for student and resident selection? *Clinical Orthopaedics and Related Research.* **378**: 115–23.

Tamblyn R *et al.* (2002) Association between licensure examination scores and practice in primary care. *Journal of the American Medical Association.* **288**(23): 3019–26.

Tunbridge M, Dickinson D and Swan P (2002) Outcomes of specialist registrar assessments. *Hospital Medicine.* **63**(11): 684–7.

Waters TM, Lefevre FV and Budetti PP (2003) Medical school attended as a predictor of medical malpractice claims. *Quality & Safety in Health Care.* **12**(5): 330–6.

Wragg A *et al.* (2003) Assessing the performance of specialist registrars. *Clinical Medicine.* **3**(2): 131–4.

Yedidia MJ *et al.* (2003) Effect of communications training on medical student performance. *Journal of the American Medical Association.* **290**(9): 1157–65.

Chapter 7

The impact of culture and climate in healthcare organisations

Michael West and Marion Spendlove

Introduction

Organisational climate and culture constitute the system of broad social contextual factors that describe the unique character of each organisation and that profoundly influence the behaviour of those who come into contact with or make up organisations. The behaviour of doctors and therefore their performance is greatly influenced by the climates and cultures of the organisations within which they do their work.

What is organisational culture?

Organisations can be described much as we might describe to our friends the experience we had in visiting a distant foreign country. We might talk about the dress, laws, physical environment, buildings, night life, recreational activities, language, humour, food, values and rituals. Similarly, organisations can be described in terms of their cultures – meanings, values, attitudes and beliefs. Surface manifestations of culture include a variety of characteristics some of which are illustrated in Box 7.1.

Box 7.1 Manifestations of culture

- **Hierarchy:** Such as how many levels from the head of the organisation to the lowest-level employee.
- **Pay levels:** High or low, whether there is performance-related pay, and what the differentials are between people at different grades.
- **Job descriptions:** How detailed or restrictive they are and what aspects they emphasise such as safety and/or patient throughput, cost savings and/or quality of patient care.
- **Informal practices:** Management and non-management employees sit at separate tables in the staff dining room; dress codes; adherence to meeting start times; involvement of patients in decisions about their care.
- **Espoused values and rituals:** An emphasis on co-operation and support versus cut-and-thrust competition between teams; cards, gifts and parties for those leaving the organisation or such events are not observed.

> - **Stories, jokes and jargon:** Commonly told stories about a particular success or the failings of management; humour about the finance department for example; and jargon or acronyms (most NHS organisations have a lexicon of acronyms and jargon and the language is often impenetrable to outsiders).
> - **Physical environment:** Waiting rooms, dining rooms, toilets. Are all spaces clean, tidy and comfortable, or is it only the areas on public display? Are there decorations such as plants and paintings and good facilities such as water fountains?

The meanings of all these aspects taken together tell us about the underlying culture of the organisation, i.e. shared meanings, values, attitudes and beliefs (Schein, 1992). Managers have been particularly interested in how to 'manage' culture and considerable resources have been spent trying to 'shape' organisational cultures and create, for example, 'a service culture', 'an open culture' or 'a people culture'.

What is organisational climate?

A closely related concept to organisational culture is 'organisational climate'. Central to most, if not all, models of organisational behaviour are employees' perceptions of the work environment, referred to generally as 'organisational climate' (Rousseau, 1988). At the broadest level, organisational climate describes how organisational members experience organisations and attach shared meanings to their perceptions of this environment (James & James, 1989). Schneider (1990) suggests that organisational climate perceptions focus on the processes, practices and behaviours that are rewarded and supported in an organisation. Most also agree that individuals interpret these aspects of the organisational environment in relation to their own sense of wellbeing (James, James & Ashe, 1990).

Individuals can describe the organisational environment both in an overall global sense as well as in a more specific, targeted manner. In relation to the global organisational environment, James and James (1989) describe four dimensions of global organisational climate, which have been identified across a number of different work contexts. These are:

1 role stress and lack of harmony (including role ambiguity, conflict and overload, subunit conflict, lack of organisational identification, and lack of management concern and awareness)
2 job challenge and autonomy (as well as job importance)
3 leadership facilitation and support (including leader trust, support, goal facilitation and interaction facilitation, and psychological and hierarchical influence) and
4 work group co-operation, friendliness, and warmth (as well as responsibility for effectiveness; James & McIntyre, 1996).

James suggests that individuals develop a global or holistic perception of their work environment (e.g. James & Jones, 1974) based on their experience in these four broad areas, which could be applied to any number of contexts, including health-care organisations.

There is uncertainty and debate about whether climate should be conceived of as a multidimensional concept or a unitary concept (Campbell *et al.*, 1970; Payne & Mansfield, 1973; James & Jones, 1974). Campbell *et al.* (1970) argue for a small number of common dimensions that constitute climate, including individual auton-omy at work, the degree of structure imposed upon people's work roles, reward orientation (positive or negative) and warmth and support. Schneider and Reichers (1983) suggest that work settings actually have many climates and they argue for the study of facet-specific climates. They believe that the choice of climate dimen-sions should be closely linked to the criteria of interests – climates are 'for some-thing', e.g. patient focus or safety, and that there is no generic organisational climate. However, most researchers believe that organisational climate can be applied as a multidimensional construct and that some dimensions are generic and applicable to most organisations. Others are unique or at least applicable to only a small range of organisations (e.g. climates for secrecy in the defence industry, or for patient care in healthcare organisations).

One orientation to the mapping of climate that has proved powerful is the Competing Values Model of organisations (Quinn & Rohrbaugh, 1981) which distinguishes between human relations, rational goals, open systems and internal process constellations of organisational values. The Competing Values approach incorporates a range of fundamental dimensions of values into a single model. It calls attention to how opposing values exist in organisations, how organisations have different mixtures of values that influence their goals, and how they go about achieving those goals. These values will be reflected in whether the organisational orientation varies more towards flexibility or control, and whether the focus of the organisation varies more towards the external or internal environment. A major theoretical strength of this model is its derivation from four orientations to the study of organisational effectiveness, reflecting long traditions in work and organisational psychology: the rational goal approach, the open systems model, the internal process approach and the human relations approach.

The rational goal approach emphasises productivity and goal achievement. The open systems model emphasises the interaction and adaptation of the organisation in its environment. The internal process approach reflects internal control of the system in order that resources are efficiently used.

Finally, the human relations approach reflects the tradition derived from socio-technical theory, emphasising the wellbeing, growth and commitment of the community of workers within the organisation. By combining these orientations into one model, Quinn and Rohrbaugh (1981) aimed to provide a broad conceptual map of the domains of organisational theory over the twentieth century. Such a map is useful:

1 in identifying the required topography of a climate measure applicable to a wide range of organisations and
2 in reflecting the means for implementing those values in terms of managerial practices, and the ends or outcomes which are emphasised or which compete in each domain.

The model does not propose that organisations will locate predominantly in one quadrant, but, reflecting the rich mix of competing views and perspectives in organisations, proposes that organisations will be active and give different emphasis to each domain.

What is the difference between culture and climate?

First, it is important to recognise that the two concepts are metaphors borrowed from quite different domains, so comparing them is rather like comparing the colour of a car with the characteristics of its engine. The first is anthropological and implies an outsider's perspective – or at least the perspective of an insider skilled in discerning elements of culture. The second is 'meteorological' and relies on the perspectives of organisational members to report on climatic conditions (it rains a lot here in England; people are supportive in this organisation). Climate is often described as members' surface experiences and perceptions, while culture shapes the meaning of events and almost unseen (and even unconscious) assumptions about how to behave in the organisation. In general, researchers agree that climate is a measure of the surface manifestations of culture and, as such, is not entirely distinct from culture. Some researchers argue that culture can only be measured by qualitative methodologies, whereas climate, as a more superficial characteristic of organisations, can be assessed using quantitative questionnaire measures.

Organisational climate measures are now widely used in public and private sector organisations to determine the prevailing climate, often being called employee attitude surveys or employee opinion surveys. One of the reasons why organisational climate surveys have become so widely used is that climate has been shown to predict organisational productivity and profitability (Patterson *et al.*, 1997; Denison, 1990), employee motivation, job satisfaction, job performance, organisational commitment and stress. For example, Patterson *et al.* (1997) found that an organisational climate oriented towards good human relations predicted 29% of the variation between companies in productivity and profitability in the UK manufacturing sector. Because of these associations between climate and performance, both researchers and practitioners continue to be interested in the concept. There is considerable debate about what aspects of climate predict what aspects of performance, partly because of the relatively weak empirical basis for the countless claims made (Wilderom, Glunk & Maslowski, 2000).

Does culture affect the performance of doctors?

By definition culture will affect the performance of doctors. To the extent that all human behaviour is profoundly influenced by the social environment, so too will doctors' performance be influenced by the norms and values embodied in the prevailing organisational culture. Although there is no direct evidence of a relationship between culture and doctors' performance, it makes sense, given what we know about the relationship between culture and behaviour, to assume that there is such a link. Researchers have focused primarily on the links between culture, climate and organisational performance and it is these associations we examine below before considering which dimensions of culture may be most likely to affect doctors' performance.

Does culture affect the performance of healthcare organisations?

Research on the links between culture and performance is not, in general, methodologically sophisticated and even the best-designed studies have produced inconsistent findings. This is at least partly due to their use of widely differing measures of climate or culture, very different outcome measures, and varying samples of organisations. Very little research has been conducted in hospital settings. One reason for this is pragmatic – hospital performance is difficult to measure. The descriptions of existing research below are selected because of their relative methodological sophistication or scale.

Argote (1989) studied 44 emergency hospital units in the United States. She analysed two dimensions of culture: the amount of agreement between professional groups about their norms (normative complementarity) and the amount of agreement existing within a group about their norms (normative consensus). The study showed that normative complementarity is positively and significantly associated with the effectiveness of emergency units, whereas the relationship between performance and normative consensus was weaker. Both were associated with promptness and quality of care.

Another study in the United States, by Aitken, Smith and Lake (1994), examined the relationship between the organisation of nursing care and mortality rates. Hospitals that were able to attract and retain good nurses and provided opportunities for good nursing care (termed 'magnet' hospitals) were compared with 195 'control' hospitals. Mortality rates, adjusted for differences in predicted mortality, were 4.6% lower in the 'magnet' hospitals than the controls. However, this study relied on the reputation of the magnet hospitals rather than more objective data.

Gerowitz *et al.* (1996) and Gerowitz (1998) used the Competing Values Framework (CVF) to classify the management team cultures of 45 Canadian hospitals, 100 UK hospitals and 120 hospitals in the USA. Measures of performance included employee loyalty, external stakeholder satisfaction, internal consistency, external resource acquisition and overall adaptability. The cultures were classified as either clan, developmental, rational or hierarchical (*see* Table 7.1). The results suggested that hospital management teams in the UK were more frequently clan and hierarchical cultures; those in the USA were more frequently rational and open cultures; and those in Canada were more often clan and rational cultures. These variations, they argue, probably reflect the political economies of the countries involved. The data suggested that the dominant culture of the management teams was significantly associated with hospital performance, but only in relation to that domain of performance valued by the culture. For example, clan cultures had higher employee loyalty; hierarchical cultures had higher internal consistency, whereas open cultures had more satisfied external stakeholders. However, the problems of direction of effects are not addressed – cultures may reflect previous performance rather than predict them or relationships may be bi-directional. Moreover, these studies mistake the original intention of the model, which proposed that organisations could not be classified into a single type but would emphasise more or less all four domains of cultural values.

Table 7.1 Characteristics of organisational cultural types

Clan	Developmental
Participative, leader as mentor, bonded by loyalty, tradition. Emphasis on morale.	Creative, adaptive, leader as risk-taker, innovator. Bonded by entrepreneurship. Emphasis on innovation.

Hierarchical	Rational
Order, rules, uniformity. Leader as administrator. Bonded by rules, policies. Emphasis on predictability.	Competitiveness. Leader as goal-orientated. Bonded by competition. Emphasis on winning.

In the most wide-ranging UK study, Mannion, Davies and Marshall (2003) conducted a national survey of 899 senior NHS managers (covering 189 acute Trusts) and linked the responses to routinely collected performance data. They also conducted in-depth case studies of six acute hospital Trusts and six primary care Trusts. The results suggested that culture did matter in that the aspects of performance stressed by the culture of the organisations were those aspects of performance on which the organisations performed best. The researchers found a significant relationship between culture, Trust characteristics and various aspects of measured (and unmeasured) performance, as well as evidence of a variety of mechanisms through which these associations may be mediated. The results suggested that performance varies in contingent ways between Trusts with different dominant cultures. Trusts with dominant clan and rational cultures were more likely to have poor quality ratings than were those with developmental cultures. Waiting times were higher in Trusts with clan, developmental and rational cultures compared to hierarchical cultures. Surveys on inpatient dignity and respect yielded higher scores in Trusts with clan cultures than in other Trusts. Staff morale was higher in clan than rational cultures. This study does not discern the likely direction of effects and it too treats the CVF as a typology into which to categorise Trusts, rather than as four continuous dimensions on which to rate Trusts.

Other evidence from the case studies in the research by Mannion, Davies and Marshall (2003) suggests a relationship between Trust leadership and performance. Apparently 'high' performing Trusts were characterised by top down 'command and control' styles of leadership. In these Trusts there was a long tradition of strong directional leadership from the centre with the senior management team setting clear and explicit performance objectives for the organisation and establishing robust internal performance management and monitoring arrangements to support these aims. High performers had clear and largely unequivocal lines of accountability. High-performing Trusts placed considerable emphasis on developing and harnessing the potential of staff to deliver the performance agenda. They also focused on recruiting and retaining staff with high commitment to a corporate rather than a purely professional agenda.

In 'low' performing Trusts, recent leaders, particularly Chief Executives, were viewed as charismatic but were generally regarded as lacking the transactional skills required to develop and maintain robust systems of performance management, and were described as being remote and disconnected from day-to-day issues in the wider organisation. Terms such as 'cabal', 'clique' and 'inner circle' were applied to senior management processes. 'Low' performing Trusts were generally characterised by an emasculated tier of middle management, and confused and fragmented systems of accountability. Human resource policies seemed to have been ignored, or were underdeveloped by the previous management regimes of the apparently 'low' performing Trusts. 'Low' performers had poor relationships with other key stakeholders and organisations within the local health economy. This extensive study provides useful guidance but is limited in its contribution by the methodological weaknesses acknowledged by the authors.

Other relevant studies have even weaker designs. Gerowitz (1998) examined the relationship between culture and performance in 120 US hospitals using managers' subjective measures of both culture and performance. Not surprisingly, given that all the data were single source and self-reported, positive associations emerged – clans and hierarchies had poor performance, and rational and open cultures had relatively good performance. Nystrom (1993) examined task norms and pragmatic values and related these to managerial ratings of performance in 13 US healthcare organisations. Again, weak but positive associations were found. Shortell *et al.* (2000) assessed the impact of Total Quality Management and culture on a wide range of outcomes for over 3000 patients across 16 hospitals undergoing coronary artery bypass grafts. Culture was assessed using the Competing Values Framework. There was little association between the predictor and outcome variables. Zimmerman *et al.* (1993) found no relationship between culture and performance in a robust study of 3672 intensive care unit (ICU) admissions involving 316 nurses and 202 doctors in nine ICUs.

None of the studies so far described offers convincing evidence of a link between culture and organisational performance in hospitals. Indeed, there is no body of strong evidence to indicate whether there is a clear relationship between culture and organisational performance in healthcare organisations. Still less is there any evidence of how culture affects doctors' performance. However, when we examine team climate as a predictor of healthcare team performance, the body of data is much stronger in substantiating a link between team climate and performance (Borrill *et al.*, 2000; 2001) than it is for the influence of organisational culture on performance.

What is the effect of employment practice on performance?

A recurring theme in the Bristol Royal Infirmary Inquiry report (Kennedy, 2001) is the importance to the provision of care for patients of how staff are managed. Over the past decade, there has been a great deal of interest in the relationship between Human Resource Management (HRM) practices and medical team performance. A number of studies have demonstrated that HRM practices, either individually or in bundles, are associated with higher levels of productivity or effectiveness at the organisational level of analysis (e.g. Arthur, 1994; d'Arcimoles, 1997; Guest & Hoque, 1994; Hoque, 1999; MacDuffie, 1995; Youndt *et al.*, 1996). A wide range of different practices has been examined in these studies. Some of the more commonly studied types of practices include staffing, training, performance appraisal, compensation, and job design. From a behavioural perspective, it has been argued that these types of practices can enhance organisational effectiveness by increasing the likelihood that employees will engage in behaviours that make a positive contribution to the organisation (Schuler & Jackson, 1987; Wright & MacMahan, 1992).

West *et al.* (2002) examined the link between the management of employees in acute hospitals (UK NHS Trusts) and outcomes such as quality of healthcare. The research was designed to determine whether there are links between HRM practices and hospital performance, as indicated by patient mortality data. The aim was to show not just whether there is a link between HRM practices, quality of care and effectiveness, but which practices affect these outcomes. The survey data were collected by telephone interviews with HR directors and chief executives, to gather information on four areas: hospital characteristics, hospital HRM strategy, employee involvement strategy and practices, and human resource management practices and procedures. Six measures of hospital performance were identified: deaths following emergency surgery, deaths following non-emergency surgery, deaths following admission for hip fractures, deaths following admission for heart attacks, re-admission rates and mortality rates, and three were employed as a reliable single factor following statistical analysis.

Controlling for a variety of possible third factors (including number of doctors per 100 beds, local health needs and prior levels of patient mortality), the study revealed a significant association between the management of employees in acute hospitals and the level of patient mortality within those hospitals. The sophistication and extensiveness of appraisal and training for hospital employees, and the percentage of staff working in teams in the hospitals, were all significantly associated with measures of patient mortality. The study provides powerful evidence that it may be possible to influence hospital performance significantly by implementing sophisticated and extensive training and appraisal systems, and encouraging a high percentage of employees to work in teams. Subsequent longitudinal research has confirmed the initial findings (West *et al.*, 2003). More research is needed to carefully examine the underlying mechanisms responsible for these associations.

To summarise, culture does appear to influence organisational performance in healthcare settings but there is too little evidence to tell us definitively which aspects of culture and climate influence which aspects of performance. However, it seems likely that domains that are given particular emphasis within an organisation will be related to the outcomes linked to those domains. One area that has received particular attention is the domain of safety.

Safety culture and safety climate

Recognition of the importance of safety culture in preventing accidents has led to numerous studies that attempt to define and assess safety culture in a number of complex, high-risk industries; Wiegmann *et al.* (2002) trace these to the nuclear accident at Chernobyl in 1986. A poor 'safety culture' was identified as a factor contributing to the disaster by the International Atomic Energy Agency (IAEA 1986, cited in Cox & Flin, 1998) and the OECD Nuclear Agency (1987, cited in Mearns & Flin, 1999; Pidgeon, 1998). Since then, safety culture has been discussed in other major accident enquiries and analyses of system failures, such as the King's

Cross Underground fire in London, and the Piper Alpha oil platform explosion in the North Sea (Cox & Flin, 1998; Pidgeon, 1998). In the UK, the report into the Bristol Royal Infirmary Inquiry (Kennedy, 2001) promoted the idea of 'creating a culture of safety', rather than a culture of fear or blame, claiming that the culture of the NHS is responsible for the lack of proactive and open management of adverse events (Kennedy, 2001).

Conceptualisations and definitions of safety culture have been derived mainly from the more general notion of organisational culture, and numerous definitions can be found in the literature. The term 'safety climate' has been used frequently, and has added to the confusion (Wiegmann *et al.*, 2002). Common themes in the definitions of safety culture include the following (Wiegmann *et al.*, 2002):

1 Safety culture is a concept defined at the group level or higher, which refers to the shared values among all the group or organisation members.
2 Safety culture is concerned with formal safety issues in an organisation, and closely related to, but not restricted to, management and supervisory systems.
3 Safety culture emphasises the contribution from everyone at every level of an organisation.
4 The safety culture of an organisation has an impact on its members' behaviour at work.
5 Safety culture is usually reflected in the contingency between reward systems and safety performance.
6 Safety culture is reflected in an organisation's willingness to develop and learn from errors, incidents, and accidents.
7 Safety culture is relatively enduring, stable and resistant to change.

Features of a safety culture in healthcare include a shared philosophy of concern, and shared responsibility for the safety of patients. 'Placing the safety of patients at the centre of the hospital's agenda is *the* crucial step towards creating and fostering a culture of safety' (Kennedy, 2001). An open and non-punitive environment, in which it is safe to admit and report adverse events, is seen as fundamental. In a safety culture, adverse events are seen as opportunities to learn and to make changes for the better, rather than an occasion to punish and forget (Kennedy, 2001).

To what extent do culture and climate factors affect the remediability of poor individual performance?

The review of the literature here makes it clear that we do not know which factors are likely to affect the remediability of poor performance by doctors and other clinical staff. One offer of help comes from a review of 'high-performance' organisational climates (Wiley & Brooks, 2000). This reports that certain dimensions of climate are associated with high performance in relation to customer satisfaction and business performance in both longitudinal and cross-sectional studies. A similar analysis would be valuable for healthcare organisations when sufficient studies have been completed but it is likely (simply in terms of face validity) that the dimensions identified by Wiley and Brooks would have some relevance for healthcare organisational performance also (*see* Box 7.2).

Box 7.2 Some key dimensions of climate/culture linked to high-performing organisations

---

Customer service
Strong emphasis on customer service
Customer problems corrected quickly
Delivers products/services in a timely fashion

Quality
Senior management demonstrates quality is a top priority
Work group quality is rated
Continuous improvement
Quality is a priority vs meeting deadlines

Involvement
Front line staff have the authority necessary to meet customers' needs
Encouragement to be innovative
Management use employees' good ideas

Training
Staff given opportunities to improve skills
Staff are satisfied with training opportunities
New employees get necessary training

Information/knowledge
Management gives clear vision/direction
Staff have a clear understanding of goals
Enough warning about changes

Teamwork/co-operation
Co-operation to get the job done
Management encourages teamwork
Problems in teams corrected quickly

Overall satisfaction
High job satisfaction
Rate the organisation as a place to work
Not seriously considering leaving the organisation

One of the most useful organisational interventions to improve healthcare in the workplace appears to be by developing effective teams. Carter and West (1999) found that team working appears to buffer health professionals against the inevitable stresses associated with the context of their work. Studies of primary care team working have found improved healthcare delivery and staff motivation (Adorian *et al.*, 1990), improved patient access to primary care (Marsh, 1991) and the deployment of skills and expertise (Marsh, 1991; Hasler, 1994). (For a more comprehensive account of the evidence on team working in organisations please see Chapter 8.) Marsh (1991) found that healthcare teams produced more cost-effective services. Other research indicates improved patient outcomes following the introduction of team working (Borrill *et al.*, 2001). However, the organisational context of healthcare is a significant barrier to team working. Historical professional divisions, status hierarchies and an organisational context within which people are not encouraged to work in teams all impede collaborative working. The key to developing effective team working within healthcare settings is to ensure that organisations are restructured and processes are changed to encourage and support team working (West & Markiewicz, 2003).

Mannion, Davies and Marshall (2003) describe a range of levers used to try to enact culture change including training and education of staff for new values and patterns of working. But this is far from an exact science and culture change programmes have not been subject to careful empirical evaluations in any settings, largely because of the large-scale requirements for longitudinal designs and the methodological challenges such evaluations pose.

Existing methods for the assessment of organisational culture and climate

There is much disagreement amongst researchers about the appropriate ways of measuring climate and culture and, within health services, most organisations have adopted their own questionnaire measures without recourse to nationally agreed measures. This has limited comparability of findings across healthcare organisations. As Mannion *et al.* (2003) point out, anyone looking for an 'ideal' instrument to measure the culture of health organisations will be disappointed. Whilst a range of instruments is available, all of them have limitations in terms of their scope, ease of use, or scientific properties. There are no simple answers to the question: Which instrument is best? The answer is that it depends on how we want to define 'culture', 'measurement' and 'organisation', the purpose of the investigation, the intended use of the results, and the availability of resources (Mannion, Davies and Marshall, 2003).

Some researchers argue for the use of multiple methods such as interviews, focus groups, observation of workplace behaviours, archival research using the documents, emails and reports arising within an organisation, along with more traditional questionnaire measures. Adopting a rigorous multi-method approach will help develop a detailed understanding of all the layers of culture within an organisation. If a value such as 'we believe in patient-centred care' emerges from an investigation, then it should trigger a search for artefacts, such as evidence of the existence of a patient participation group, and also a search for tacit assumptions, such as the expectation that this value is shared amongst everyone who works in the organisations (Mannion, Davies & Marshall, 2003). However, such multi-method approaches are difficult to integrate and expensive in practice. Despite the debates about the appropriate methods for assessing culture and climate, most commentators (e.g. Ashkanasy, Broadfoot & Falkus, 2000) agree that quantitative questionnaires are an appropriate and convenient way of assessing culture and climate. The difficulty is in the choice of measure (see for example Ashkanasy, Broadfoot & Falkus, 2000).

Attitude surveys offer an opportunity to measure the degree of transparency and open communication being fostered by patient-safety projects, and are common in the airline industry (Helmreich & Merritt, 1998; Sexton, Thomas & Helmreich, 2000). These have shown a direct relationship between pilot attitude and unsafe flying conditions. The surveys have been modified for use in healthcare and there are clear indications that provider attitude may be correlated with patient morbidity and mortality (Shortell *et al.*, 1994; Sexton, Thomas & Helmreich, 2000).

Hill & West (2003) produced a climate measure for UK healthcare organisations that is based on a larger instrument with excellent psychometric properties including predictive validity for organisational performance (Hill & West, 2003; Patterson *et al.*, 2003).

Possibly the most convenient and potentially informative measure for the assessment of climate/culture would be the new annual NHS National Staff Survey instrument Commission for Health Improvement 2004. This survey will enable NHS organisations, for the first time, to be benchmarked against other, similar NHS organisations and the NHS as a whole, on a range of measures of staff satisfaction and opinion.

Empirical efforts to study safety culture and its relationship to organisational outcomes have remained unsystematic, fragmented and underspecified in theoretical terms (Pidgeon, 1998). Surveys and questionnaires have been widely used to assess safety culture within a variety of industries. There are no standardised 'off the shelf' tools that can be used across domains, or even within a single domain (Cox & Flin, 1998), and both quantitative and qualitative methods are used.

One of the major questions to consider in the development of tools for assessing safety culture is whether the assessment should be at global or local levels. Should the organisation as a whole be assessed (global) or do assessments need to occur within the organisation's various sublevels, such as divisions or departments (local)? Some researchers (Reason, 1997; Helmreich & Merritt, 1998) have suggested that cultures vary considerably across operational settings such as the flight deck, maintenance and ramp environments. The same is likely to be true across various departments within other types of organisations as well. Separate assessment instruments may be needed to examine the different units within an organisation (Wiegmann *et al.*, 2002; Pizzi, Goldfarb & Nash, 2001). Note also that there are no direct data supporting the effect of promoting a culture of safety. The contribution of culture to safety relative to other causal factors is also unknown.

Factors for which early intervention is effective as a preventive measure

There exists a variety of hard indicators of cultures that are likely to lead to poor performance. Features of poor performance include high levels of turnover and intention to quit, high levels of sickness absence and high levels of errors, accidents and incidents at work. Other measures include low levels of satisfaction and high levels of stress. These standard indicators of organisational health can be used to monitor underlying cultural or climate problems and suggest the need for early intervention. By monitoring climate and culture annually as well as gathering data on the hard indicators, it is possible to identify changes in culture/climate associated with changes in levels of absenteeism, turnover and accidents. This should be possible, given the application of an annual staff survey in the NHS and the routine collection of data on absenteeism and turnover.

Conclusion

On the surface, the links between the culture of an organisation and the performance of individuals seem to be obvious. Indeed, it would go against the whole notion of culture to argue that doctors' performance was not directly and powerfully affected by the culture of the organisations of which they are a part. Yet close examination of the evidence reveals that many studies that link organisational culture with performance do not stand close scrutiny. It is not possible to cite studies that directly link organisational culture with the performance of doctors, or, indeed, with any other group of individuals. Lack of methodological rigour and sophistication of design, absence of standardised objective measures for culture and performance, and the small number of studies conducted in hospital settings mean that these links remain obscure.

There are indications that domains of cultural emphasis will be related to the outcomes linked to those domains. Thus a safety climate may be related to lower levels of accidents; a patient-centred culture will be associated with higher levels of patient satisfaction. It is possible that particular dominant cultures can influence certain aspects of performance, but it is unclear which aspects of culture and climate influence which aspects of performance. Furthermore, such relationships may be bi-directional, as performance itself is equally likely to affect organisational culture. In short, the literature on organisational culture and performance is suggestive, but inconclusive.

Yet some studies of particular aspects of culture allow us to draw a few tentative conclusions. For example, there is evidence of the importance of certain HRM practices in healthcare, such as working in teams. Such studies shed some light on which practices affect which aspects of performance although, again, the underlying mechanisms are unclear. What is needed is research that focuses on the key outcome variables and identifies the elements and dimensions of culture and climate that are likely to be related. These links can then be studied in depth. The results of the 2003 NHS National Staff Survey will offer a rich source of preliminary data for analysing culture and performance in healthcare, and data about the culture that doctors work in can be measured against different aspects of their performance. It will then be possible to understand more about how organisational climate and culture influence their performance.

References

Adorian D *et al*. (1990) Group discussions with the health care team: a method of improving care of hypertension in general practice. *Journal of Human Hypertension*. 4(3): 265–8.

Aitken LH, Smith HL and Lake ET (1994) Lower Medicare mortality among a set of hospitals known for good nursing care. *Medical Care*. 32(8): 771–87.

Argote L (1989) Agreement about norms and work-unit effectiveness: evidence from the field. *Basic and Applied Social Psychology*. 10(2): 131–40.

Arthur JB (1994) Effects of human resource systems on manufacturing performance and turnover. *Academy of Management Journal*. 37(3): 670–87.

Ashkanasy NM, Broadfoot LE and Falkus S (2000) Questionnaire measures of organizational culture. In: NM Ashkanasy, CPM Wilderom and MF Peterson (eds) *Handbook of Organizational Culture and Climate*. Sage, Thousand Oaks, CA, pp. 131–45.

Borrill CS *et al*. (2001) *The Effectiveness of Health Care Teams in the National Health Service*. University of Aston, Birmingham.

Borrill C *et al.* (2000) Team working and effectiveness in health care. *British Journal of Health Care Management.* **6**: 364–71.

Campbell JP *et al.* (1970) *Managerial Behaviour, Performance and Effectiveness.* McGraw Hill, New York.

Carter A and West MA (1999) Sharing the burden: teamwork in health care settings. In: J Firth-Cozens and R Payne (eds) *Stress in Health Professionals: psychological and organisational causes and interventions.* John Wiley & Sons, Chichester, pp. 191–202.

Cox S and Flin R (1998) Safety culture: philosopher's stone or man of straw? *Work and Stress.* **12**(3): 189–201.

d'Arcimoles CH (1997) Human resource policies and company performance: a quantitative approach using longitudinal data. *Organization Studies.* **18**(5): 857–74.

Denison DR (1990) *Corporate Culture and Organizational Effectiveness.* John Wiley & Sons, New York.

Gerowitz MB (1998) Do TQM interventions change management culture? Findings and implications. *Quality Management in Health Care.* **6**(3): 1–11.

Gerowitz MB *et al.* (1996) Top management culture and performance in Canadian, UK and US hospitals. *Health Services Management Research.* **9**(2): 69–78.

Guest D and Hoque K (1994) The good, the bad and the ugly: employee relations in new non-union workplaces. *Human Resource Management Journal.* **5**: 1–14.

Hasler J (1994) *The Primary Care Team.* Royal Society of Medicine Press, London.

Helmreich RL and Merritt AC (1998) *Culture at Work in Aviation and Medicine: national, organizational and professional influences.* Ashgate, Brookfield, VT.

Hill F and West MA (2003) *Is Organisational Climate a Meaningful Construct?* Aston Business School Working Paper Series, Birmingham.

Hoque K (1999) Human resource management and performance in the UK hotel industry. *British Journal of Industrial Relations.* **37**(3): 419–43.

James LA and James LR (1989) Integrating work environment perceptions: explorations into the measurement of meaning. *Journal of Applied Psychology.* **74**(5): 739–51.

James LR and Jones AP (1974) Organizational climate: review of theory and research. *Psychological Bulletin.* **81**(12): 1096–112.

James LR, James LA and Ashe DK (1990) The meaning of organizations: the role of cognition and values. In: B Schneider (ed.) *Organizational Climate and Culture.* Jossey-Bass, San Francisco, pp. 40–84.

James LR and McIntyre MD (1996) Perceptions of organizational climate. In: KR Murphy (ed.) *Individual Differences and Behavior in Organizations.* Jossey-Bass, San Francisco, pp. 416–50.

Kennedy L (2001) *Learning from Bristol: the report of the Public Inquiry into children's heart surgery at the Bristol Royal Infirmary 1984–1995.* Final Report [online]. The Stationery Office, London. Available at: www.bristol-inquiry.org.uk [Accessed 8 October 2004].

MacDuffie JP (1995) Human-resource bundles and manufacturing performance: organizational logic and flexible production systems in the world auto industry. *Industrial & Labor Relations Review.* **48**(2): 197–221.

Mannion R, Davies HTO and Marshall MD (2003) Cultures for performance in health care: evidence of the relationship between organisational culture and organisational performance in the NHS. York Centre for Health Economics, York.

Marsh GN (1991) Caring for larger lists. *BMJ.* **303**(6813): 1312–16.

Mearns KJ and Flin R (1999) Assessing the state of organisational safety: culture or climate? *Current Psychology: Developmental, Learning, Personality, Social.* **18**(1): 5–17.

Nystrom PC (1993) Organisational cultures, strategies, and commitments in health care organizations. *Health Care Management Review.* **18**(1): 43–9.

Patterson MG, West MA, Lawthom RL and Nickell S (1997) *People Management and Business Performance.* Institute for Personnel and Development, London.

Payne RL and Mansfield R (1973) Relationships of perceptions of organizational climate to organizational structure, context and hierarchical position. *Administrative Science Quarterly.* **18**(4): 515–26.

Pidgeon N (1998) Safety culture: key theoretical issues. *Work and Stress.* **12**(3): 202–16.

Pizzi LT, Goldfarb NI and Nash DB (2001) Promoting a culture of safety. In: KG Shojania *et al.* (eds) *Making Health Care Safer: a critical analysis of patient safety practices.* Evidence Report/Technology Assessment No. 43. Agency for Healthcare Research and Quality, Rockville, MD, pp. 447–57.

Quinn RE and Rohrbaugh J (1981) A competing values approach to organisational effectiveness. *Public Productivity Review.* **5**: 122–40.

Reason J (1997) *Managing the Risks of Organisational Accidents.* Ashgate, Aldershot.

Rousseau DM (1988) The construction of climate in organizational research. In: CL Cooper and IT Robinson (eds) *International Review of Industrial and Organizational Psychology.* John Wiley & Sons, Chichester, pp. 139–58.

Schein EH (1992) *Organisational Culture and Leadership* (2e). Jossey Bass Wiley, San Francisco.

Schneider B (1990) The climate for service: an application of the climate construct. In: B Schneider (ed.) *Organizational Climate and Culture.* Jossey-Bass, San Francisco, pp. 383–412.

Schneider B and Reichers AE (1983) On the etiology of climates. *Personnel Psychology.* **36**(1): 19–39.

Schuler RS and Jackson SE (1987) Linking competitive strategies with human resource management practices. *Academy of Management Executive.* **1**(3): 207–19.

Sexton JB, Thomas EJ and Helmreich RL (2000) Error, stress and teamwork in medicine and aviation: cross sectional surveys. *BMJ.* **320**(7237): 745–9.

Shortell SM *et al.* (2000) Assessing the impact of Total Quality Management and organisational culture on multiple outcomes of care for coronary artery bypass graft surgery patients. *Medical Care.* **38**(2): 201–17.

Shortell SM *et al.* (1994) The performance of intensive care units: does good management make a difference? *Medical Care.* **32**(5): 508–25.

West MA *et al.* (2003) *The Relationship between Staff Management Practices and Patient Mortality in Acute Hospitals: a longitudinal study.* Aston Business School Working Paper Series, Birmingham.

West MA *et al.* (2002) The link between the management of employees and patient mortality in acute hospitals. *International Journal of Human Resource Management.* **13**(8): 1299–310.

West MA and Markiewicz L (2003) *Building Team-based Working: a practical guide to organizational transformation.* Blackwell, Oxford.

Wiegmann DA *et al.* (2002) *A Synthesis of Safety Culture and Safety Climate Research.* Technical Report ARL-02-3-FAA-02-2 prepared for Federal Aviation Administration, Atlantic City International Airport, NJ. Aviation Research Lab Institute of Aviation, Illinois.

Wilderom CPM, Glunk U and Maslowski R (2000) Organizational culture as a predictor of organizational performance. In: NM Ashkanasy, CPM Wilderom and MF Peterson (eds) *Handbook of Organizational Culture and Climate.* Sage, Thousand Oaks, CA, pp. 193–209.

Wiley JW and Brooks SM (2000) The high-performance organizational climate: how workers describe top-performing units. In: NM Ashkanasy, CPM Wilderom and MF Peterson (eds) *Handbook of Organizational Culture and Climate.* Sage, Thousand Oaks, CA, pp. 177–92.

Wright PM and McMahan GC (1992) Theoretical perspectives for strategic human resource management. *Journal of Management.* **18**(2): 295–320.

Youndt MA *et al.* (1996) Human resource management, manufacturing strategy, and firm performance. *Academy of Management Journal.* **39**(4): 836–66.

Zimmerman J *et al.* (1993) Improving intensive care: observations based on organizational case studies in nine intensive care units: a prospective multicenter study. *Critical Care Medicine.* **21**(10): 1443–51.

Chapter 8

The influence of team working

Michael West and Carol Borrill

Teams are a particular form of work group. They are groups of people who share responsibility for producing products or delivering services. They share overall work objectives and ideally have the necessary authority, autonomy and resources to achieve these objectives. Team members are dependent on each other to achieve the objectives and therefore have to work closely, interdependently and supportively to achieve the team's goals. Members have distinct and clear roles. Effective teams have as few members as necessary to perform the task. And the team is recognised by others in the organisation as a team (West *et al.*, 2003).

It is important that initially teams are defined by their task not by the team members. Team members are selected because they have the mix of skills necessary for the task to be completed successfully. Moreover, team members work interdependently rather than in parallel. Their interaction influences task performance and therefore team members should be skilled in and assessed against effective interaction with other team members.

Teamwork is a core part of the delivery of health services, whether in well-defined senior management teams, loosely knit community teams who come together only for team meetings, or relatively long-term theatre teams where some staff, like trainee doctors or bank nurses, come and go but the core team continues. Nevertheless, defining a health service team is not always easy: the boundaries of a theatre team stretch into sterile services, portering, intensive therapy units, for example (Firth-Cozens, 1998). Moreover, it contains within it teams which may define themselves by their professional group as well as by the task; for example, theatre nursing teams. Although looking at the evidence on teamwork from outside of healthcare is useful – particularly as group dynamics are largely universal – we need to remember the special characteristics and difficulties faced by healthcare teams.

To what extent are team-based working and effective teamwork associated with organisational performance?

Team-based working refers to the extent to which organisations are structured around teams and the extent to which employees work in real (as opposed to nominal) teams. Effective teamwork describes the extent to which teams perform effectively and is usually assessed by team productivity, including quality, innovation, team member satisfaction and team viability. (Can the team continue to work together effectively?)

Reduced hospitalisation and costs

Sommers *et al.* (2000) compared primary healthcare teams in the US with physician care across 18 private practices, and concluded that teams lowered hospitalisation rates and reduced physician visits while maintaining function for elderly patients with chronic illness and functional deficits. Significant cost savings came from reduced hospitalisation, which more than accounted for the costs of setting up the team and making regular home visits. Jones (1992) also reported that families that received care from a primary healthcare team had fewer hospitalisations, fewer operations, fewer physician visits for illness and more physician visits for health supervision than control families. A similar pattern emerged for terminally ill patients, where their increased utilisation of home care services were more than offset by average savings of 18% in hospital costs (Hughes *et al.*, 1992).

Improved service provision

Nurses in England reported that working together in primary healthcare teams reduced duplication, streamlined patient care and enabled specialist skills to be used more cost-effectively (Ross, Rink & Furne, 2000). Jansson, Isacsson and Lindholm (1992) analysed the records of general practitioners and other district carers over 6 years in Sweden. Care teams (GP, district nurse, assistant nurse) were introduced into one region but not in another comparative region. The care teams reported a large rise in the overall number of patient contacts and in the proportion of the population who accessed the district nurse, but a reduction in emergency visits, which they attributed to better accessibility to, and continuity of care from, the teams. Jackson *et al.* (1993) reported a similar pattern 12 months after the introduction of a community mental health team in England.

Team working also contributes to performance in healthcare organisations by reducing errors and improving the quality of patient care. The association between team working and these aspects of performance is reported in a number of studies (Reith, 1998; Firth-Cozens, 1998; Adorian *et al.*, 1990).

Poor teamwork has been shown to predict early retirement (Luce *et al.*, 2002) and increased sickness absence in doctors (Kivimaki *et al.*, 2001).

Lower patient mortality

West *et al.* (2002) examined the relationship between the people management practices in hospitals and patient mortality and found a strong relationship between Human Resource Management practices and patient mortality. The higher the percentage of staff working in teams in hospitals, the lower the patient mortality. On average, in hospitals where over 60% of staff worked in formal teams, mortality was around 5% lower than would be expected.

The study controlled for a variety of factors that might influence the results including number of doctors, variations in local health profiles, hospital income, etc. The study demonstrated that the effects were from HRM practices to mortality rather than vice versa.

Enhanced patient satisfaction

Hughes *et al.* (1992) compared the provision of hospital-based team home care and customary care for 171 terminally ill patients in a large US Department of Veterans Affairs hospital. Both patients and caregivers expressed significantly higher levels of satisfaction with continuous and comprehensive care, at one month, and they continued to express higher levels of satisfaction at 6 months (Sommers *et al.*, 2000). The most capable teams were reported to have provided superior levels of quality care.

Staff motivation and wellbeing

Stress levels are relatively high in doctors (Firth-Cozens, 2001). For example, Houston & Allt (1997) found that insomnia, stress and error rates increased when junior doctors began new posts. However, there is evidence that team-based working leads to lower stress. Wall *et al.* (1997) found that 28% of health staff were above threshold on the General Health Questionnaire compared to 18% of workers in the British Household Panel Survey of 1993.

Within the NHS, fewer staff working in 'real' teams – ones with clearly defined roles, whose members worked together to achieve them, with different roles for different members, and recognised externally as a functional team (21%) – had higher stress levels than those in teams which did not meet these criteria (30%). Those not working in teams had the highest levels of all (35%) (Carter and West, 1999). These differences between types of team membership in stress levels were accounted for by the higher levels of social support and role clarity experienced by those working in clearly defined teams. Similarly, primary care team working has been reported to improve staff motivation and satisfaction (Wood, Farrow & Elliott, 1994).

West and Anderson (1996) carried out a longitudinal study of the functioning of top management teams in 27 UK hospitals and examined relationships between team and organisational factors and hospital innovation. Their results showed that top team processes best predicted the overall level of innovation in the hospitals, while the proportion of innovative team members predicted the rated radicalness of innovations introduced. West and Wallace (1991) found that team collaboration, commitment and tolerance of diversity were positively related to team innovativeness.

To what extent does working in a team influence a doctor's performance?

Early studies of organisational behaviour showed that work groups profoundly influenced individual behaviour. In the 1920s and 1930s, several studies were carried out at Western Electric's Hawthorne Works in Chicago to examine the factors that affected workers' performance. The results suggested that the characteristics of the social setting or group in which behaviour takes place are at least as important as the technical aspects of the work in explaining performance. The Hawthorne studies (Roethlisberger & Dixon, 1939) established how group influences have a major impact on work group behaviour and subsequent research has consistently and convincingly demonstrated the profound influence that group or team membership has on the behaviour and performance of individuals (for excellent reviews see Brown, 2000; Hackman, 1992). These influences can be both benign (social facilitation, improved decision making) and malign (conformity, group polarisation) (West, Tjosvold & Smith, 2003).

What aspects of teamwork are most likely to influence a doctor's performance?

Much effort has been devoted to understanding factors which promote group effectiveness, and the thinking of most researchers has been dominated by an input-process-output model, mainly because of its simplicity and utility (*see* Figure 8.1).

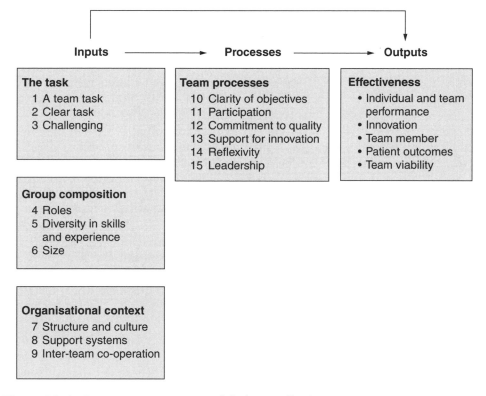

Figure 8.1 An input-process-output model of team effectiveness.

Inputs

Clear, challenging team task

One of the most influential models of task classification, proposed by Hackman and colleagues (Hackman, 1990; Hackman & Lawler, 1971; Hackman & Oldham, 1975) identifies five characteristics of motivating tasks: autonomy, task variety, task significance, task identity and relevant task feedback. Variations in these characteristics are related to both job satisfaction (Drory & Shamir, 1988; Hackman & Lawler, 1971) and work group and individual effectiveness.

Within health service work, particularly in secondary care, many of these factors remain. However, in primary care, general practitioners are increasingly concerned that most of them are being eroded, influencing their decisions to retire early (Newton *et al.*, 2004).

For a team and its members to be effective, the team must have clear objectives that fit with the overall objectives of the wider organisation. In turn, individual team members must have clear objectives that contribute to the overall objectives of the team as a whole. The task of the team must be a task that is better performed by a team rather than a group of individuals working in parallel. Many ward teams are simply nurses working together in the same physical location without a high level of interdependent work (Mathieu, Marks & Zaccaro, 2001; West *et al.*, 2003; West & Markiewicz, 2003).

Group composition: diversity

There is remarkable agreement that heterogeneity of skills in teams performing complex tasks, such as the delivery of healthcare, is good for effectiveness (e.g. Campion *et al.*, 1993; Guzzo & Dickson, 1996; Jackson, 1996; Milliken & Martins, 1996; Borrill *et al.*, 2000, 2001). Heterogeneity of skills and knowledge implies that each team member brings a different perspective to the problem, a necessary ingredient for creative solutions (Paulus & Nijstad, 2003; West *et al.*, 2002).

Teams that are diverse in task-related attributes are often diverse in individual attributes. Individual characteristics can trigger stereotypes and prejudice (Jackson, 1996) which, via interteam conflict (Tajfel, 1978; Tajfel & Turner, 1979; Hogg & Abrams, 1988), can affect team processes and outcomes. As an example, Alexander *et al.* (1996) summarised that individuals in multidisciplinary treatment teams in US Department of Veterans Affairs hospitals who were members of larger and more heterogeneous teams had lower perceptions of team functioning than those in smaller, less diverse teams. The greater the diversity of individual characteristics of team tenure, age and occupation within teams, the more negatively team members assessed team functioning.

However, none of these studies relate to patient outcomes, and inevitably heterogeneous teams are necessary for patient care (Jenkins, Fallowfield & Poole, 2001).

Another approach suggests that diversity should be developed within teams because it encourages innovation. For example, in a study of 100 primary health-care teams, Borrill *et al.* (2000) found that the greater the number of professional groups represented in the team, the higher the levels of innovation in patient care. Groups that contain people with diverse *and* overlapping knowledge domains and skills are particularly creative (Dunbar, 1997). Diversity of functional backgrounds may also improve team performance as a result of the higher level of external communication that team members initiate, because of their functional diversity. In short, doctors working in multidisciplinary teams are more likely to have their views challenged, their creativity stimulated and the quality of their decision making improved.

Diversity also has a downside. When diversity begins to threaten the group's safety and integration, effectiveness and innovation implementation may suffer. The challenge is to create sufficient diversity within the team without threatening their shared view of their task and their ability to communicate and work effectively together.

Diversity of knowledge and skills is beneficial for team performance and innovation if group processes minimise losses due to disagreements, misunderstandings and suspicion arising from diversity of perspectives (West *et al.*, 2002).

Age

People are more likely to leave teams composed of people of different ages than teams that are homogeneous with respect to age. Moreover, age-diverse top management teams ran companies that were subsequently less profitable (West, Patterson & Dawson, 1999).

Gender

Gender is an important influence on communication within teams. Not only are men consistently more assertive in public situations and confrontations (Kimble, Marsh & Kiska, 1984; Mathison & Tucker, 1982), but also communication expectations differ for men and women. Stereotypical women are passive, submissive and expressive communicators, while men are expected to be active, controlling and less expressive (LaFrance & Mayo, 1978). Punishment for violation of expectations (Jussim, 1986; Jussim, Coleman & Lerch, 1987; Jackson *et al.*, 1993) may influence both the perceptions of women in teams and their willingness to participate in team communication. Such considerations are vitally important in healthcare teams where women dominate in number but men predominate in the highest status positions. As women increasingly become leaders of clinical teams they may need different forms of leadership training.

There is some evidence that the more women there are in a team (excluding women-only teams), the more positively do all team members report the team's functioning. This may be because women focus more on the participation and involvement of their colleagues, whereas men are more likely to focus on the task (Eagly & Johnson, 1990). Moreover, men are more likely to interrupt women in team meetings and to pay less attention to their contributions (West, Borrill & Unsworth, 1998).

There is also increasing evidence from studies in a variety of sectors in the USA that the longer teams are together, the better they tend to perform (Hackman, 2002). This makes sense, since the longer they work together, the more they come to have a clear understanding of each other's styles of working and strengths.

The longer a team spends together, the lower the team error rate as the team learns to compensate for individual errors (Foushee & Helmreich, 1988). This is important in clinical teams where young doctors are peripatetic during their training, while senior clinicians see themselves as 'here for the duration', particularly compared to those in management. These differences in tenure also have an effect on the reporting of errors.

Culture

Does cultural diversity enable or hinder team performance? This is not a simple question to answer, but in one of the very few longitudinal studies in this area,

Watson, Kumar and Michaelsen (1993) found that groups that were hetero-geneous with respect to culture initially performed more poorly on a series of business case exercises than culturally homogeneous groups. As group members gained experience with each other over time, however, performance differences between culturally homogeneous and heterogeneous groups largely disappeared and more recent evidence suggests that heterogeneous teams outperform homo-geneous teams (West, Tjosvold & Smith, 2003).

Group composition: team size

Since bigger teams experience much greater strains on effective communication, in most sectors teams tend to be divided once they reach 12 or 13 members. But primary and secondary healthcare teams can have 20, 30 or 40 members. These 'teams' are more correctly termed 'organisations'. Hackman (2002), whose work represents some of the most in-depth explorations of team effectiveness, suggests that teams should consist of the minimum number of members necessary to get the job done and no more than six to eight people. However, this is likely to be unrealistic in most health service teams. The performance of doctors working in larger teams may therefore be inhibited, and the performance of doctors working in teams of appropriate size enhanced.

Organisational context

Structure and culture

There is growing evidence that the performance of teams and their members is affected by the organisational context (Hackman, 1990; Hackman, 2002; Mathieu, Marks & Zaccaro, 2001). Teamwork is more likely to fail if organisational systems are geared towards managing individuals. Creating team-based organisations means flattening the structure, changing the support systems and developing a team-based, supportive culture (see West & Markiewicz, 2003 for a detailed account of the processes involved and also Chapter 7). Instead of focusing on the management of individual performance, as in most organisations, the focus is on team function and effectiveness.

However, rewarding teams for excellence is difficult in the health service, where pay differentials are wide. It is often the consultant who gets the merit award for a team's success (Firth-Cozens, 2001).

Support systems

Hackman (1990) concluded that there are six areas within which teams need organisational support: targets, resources, information, education, feedback and technical/process assistance in functioning. Examining the extent to which organ-isations provide team support in these areas can help in discovering the underlying causes of team and team member performance difficulties.

1 **Targets:** Teams need support from an organisation to determine their targets or objectives. Surprisingly few teams receive clear targets from their organisations, often because organisational targets and aims are not sufficiently clear (West & Poulton, 1995).

2 **Resources:** The organisation must provide adequate resources to enable the team to achieve its targets or objectives.

3 **Information:** Teams need information from the organisation that will enable them to achieve their targets and objectives. If teams are not told about changes in strategy or policy, they will not function effectively.

4 **Education:** Organisations must provide the appropriate education for staff to enable team members to contribute most effectively to team functioning and to develop as individuals.

5 **Feedback:** To function effectively, teams require timely and appropriate organisational feedback on their performance. Many healthcare teams do not receive such feedback. This is highly likely to have deleterious effects on team and individual doctors' performance.

6 **Technical and process assistance:** Organisations must provide the specialised knowledge and technical support to enable teams to perform their work effectively. For example, a primary healthcare team engaged in developing practice objectives by identifying the health needs of the practice population might need advice on how and where to gather data. Process assistance refers to the organisational help provided when teams encounter process problems, such as intense interpersonal difficulties.

Inter-group co-operation

Cohesive, effective teams may become more competitive in relation to other teams precisely because they have been developed so effectively. Good team-based working ensures that norms of interteam co-operation are established from the beginning and reinforced throughout the process. This in turn enhances the effectiveness of the team and its members (see Mathieu, Marks & Zaccaro, 2001).

Developing shared objectives

Goal-setting research indicates that clarity of team objectives facilitates team and team member performance (Locke & Latham, 1991). Where doctors do not share a commitment to a set objectives or goals, disagreement leads to disintegration, lack of safety, diversity and inhibited team performance.

Participation in decision making

Effective communication amongst team members with shared decision making leads to effective decision making, creativity and innovation. In general, high participation in decision making means less resistance to change and therefore greater likelihood of effectiveness and innovation.

Several research studies in England have highlighted the causes and consequences of interprofessional communication problems within primary healthcare teams (West & Field, 1995). Some healthcare teams failed to set aside time for regular meetings to define objectives, clarify roles, apportion tasks, encourage participation and handle change. Other reasons for poor communication included differences in status, power, educational background, assertiveness of members of the team, and the assumption that the doctors will be the leaders. The authors argued that joint professional training and the instigation of regular team meetings were necessary to promote good communication.

Researchers have highlighted the impact of communication problems on patients across different types of teams. Nievaard's (1987) work in two general hospitals in the Netherlands demonstrated the phenomenon of problem shifting, where communication problems within the team were transferred onto patients. Yeatts and Seward (2000) reported similar findings in a US rural nursing home, concluding that enhanced communication between team members positively affected the service to residents. Observations of a high performing team's meetings showed that team members had a high level of respect for each other. They listened to each other, and were not afraid to disagree when they held different views. Team members sought and valued approval from each other, and they assisted each other to complete tasks.

Emphasis on quality of patient care

Discussion of competing perspectives is fundamental to the generation of effective decision making, creativity and innovation (Mumford & Gustafson, 1988; Nemeth & Owens, 1996; Tjosvold, 1998). Task-related conflict (as opposed to destructive relationship conflicts – see DeDreu, 1997) arises from a common concern with the quality of task performance in relation to shared objectives. Task conflict includes the appraisal of, and constructive challenges to, the team's performance. Team members are more committed to effective and excellent performance than they are to bland consensus or personal victory.

Dean Tjosvold and colleagues have presented cogent arguments and strong supportive evidence that such constructive (task-related) controversy in a co-operative group improves the quality of decision making and creativity of individual practitioners and the team overall (Tjosvold, 1991). Constructive controversy is characterised by full exploration of opposing opinions and frank analyses of task-related issues. It occurs when decision-makers believe they work in a co-operative group, where mutually beneficial goals are emphasised, rather than in a competitive context; where they feel their personal competence is confirmed rather than questioned; and where they perceive processes of mutual influence rather than attempted dominance.

DeDreu and De Vries (1997) suggest that a homogeneous workforce, in which dissent is suppressed by power, hierarchy or professional hegemony, reduces effectiveness, innovation, individuality and independence of thinking (DeDreu & De Vries, 1993; see also Nemeth & Nemeth-Brown, 2003). Disagreement about ideas on patient care within a team can be beneficial. Task-related conflict may lead team members to re-evaluate the status quo and adapt their objectives, strategies or processes more appropriately to their situation. However, DeDreu and Weingart (2003) find that high levels of conflict within teams, regardless of whether the conflict is focused on relationships or tasks, inhibits team member and team effectiveness and innovation.

Support for innovation

Innovation is more likely to occur in groups where there is support for innovation, and where innovative attempts are rewarded rather than punished (Amabile, 1983;

Kanter, 1983; West, 1990). In a longitudinal study of 27 hospital top management teams, support for innovation was the most powerful predictor of team innovation of any of the group processes so far discussed (West & Anderson, 1996). In general, there are significant positive relationships between healthcare team effectiveness and team innovation, as in most other sectors (Borrill *et al.*, 2000).

Reflexivity

Team reflexivity is the extent to which team members collectively reflect upon the team's objectives, strategies and processes as well as the wider organisation and environment, and adapt accordingly (West, 2000). This is particularly important in terms of the cultural change outlined in *An Organisation with a Memory* (Department of Health, 2000). Reflexivity requires care, however, since reflection is likely to reveal gaps between how the team is performing and how it would like to perform. Edmondson's work (1996; 1999) helps us to understand the conditions which encourage reflexivity and learning. She found major differences between newly formed intensive care nursing teams in their management of medication errors. In some teams, members openly acknowledged and discussed their medication errors (giving too much or too little of a drug, or administering the wrong drug) and discussed ways to avoid their occurrence. In others, members kept information about errors to themselves. Learning about the causes of errors, and devising innovation to prevent future errors were only possible in teams of the former type. Edmondson argues that learning and innovation only take place where group members trust each other's intentions and believe that well-intentioned action will not lead to punishment or rejection; Edmondson calls this 'team safety'. The term is meant to suggest a realistic, learning-oriented attitude to effort, error and change – not to a careless sense of permissiveness, or an unrelentingly positive affect. Safety is not the same as comfort (1999: 14).

Leadership

- Personalities of leaders, including agreeableness and emotional stability, plus intelligence, self-confidence, determination, integrity and sociability.
- Decision-making style.
- Leadership style.

Attitudes to safety

The team leader has three overall tasks to perform: to create the conditions that enable the team to do its job; to build and maintain the team as a performing unit; and to coach and support the team to success (see Hackman, 2002 for an extended and excellent exploration of these three tasks). First, creating the right conditions means ensuring that the team has a clear task to perform and making sure that the team has the resources it needs to do its work. It is also important for the leader to define the team's boundaries. Some healthcare teams are composed of core members who work together every day and have others who join the team (such as medical oncologists in breast cancer care teams). The team is its core members. The peripheral members work with the team from time to time but cannot operate as full team members because they are not together enough with the others. Second, in order to build and maintain the team as a performing unit the leader must ensure that the team consists of members with the necessary skills and abilities. The team must be sufficiently diverse. Third, the team leader must coach and support the team to success. This means intervening to help the team do its work successfully by giving direction and support. The importance of leadership in producing safer care is outlined in Chapter 9 of this book.

Much of the research on team leadership has focused on the contribution made by a single leader. However, leadership can also be provided by one or more individuals who are either formally appointed to the role, or emerge from within the team. Irrespective of the team type and team task, team members should be clear about who is in this role. West *et al.* (2003) found that leadership clarity is associated with clear team objectives, high levels of participation, commitment to excellence and support for innovation.

Leaders of healthcare teams must be trained in the skills and competences required of team leaders (Hackman, 2002; Firth-Cozens, 2004; West *et al.*, 2003).

Which of these factors is most influential?

In order to answer this question we identify the key factors associated with the failure of team working and team-based organisations:

Teams without tasks

The only point of having a team is to get a job done. The tasks that teams perform should be tasks that are best performed by a team. Building teams for their own sake is likely to damage organisational functioning and encourage conflict, anger and disruption (West & Markiewicz, 2003).

Teams without freedom and responsibility

Creating teams and then failing to give them the freedom and authority to make decisions and allow them to accomplish their tasks in the most effective way is a common failing in healthcare organisations. Teams are created but not given the power to make decisions, implement them and bring about change. Often, the number of layers in the organisational hierarchy barely changes. Consequently, expectations are not met and team members lose faith in the concept of teamwork other than as a comfortable concept of members being supportive to each other.

Organisations deeply structured around individuals

Teams are set up in many places in the organisation but all the systems are geared towards managing individuals. Creating team-based organisations means radically altering the structure, the support systems and the culture.

Team leaders or supervisors

Team leadership is very different from traditional supervision. Supervisors are often directive rather than facilitative. They give advice rather than seek it. They try to determine views rather than integrate them, and play a directive rather than a supportive role. The function of a team leader is very different – it is to ensure that the team profits optimally from its shared knowledge, experience and skills.

Some people have greater aptitude for leadership roles than others.

Strong teams in conflict

Teams can become rigidly defended silos. Cohesive, effective teams may become competitive and discriminatory in relation to other teams precisely because they have developed effectively. Good team-based working ensures that norms of interteam co-operation are established from the beginning and reinforced throughout the process.

Team composition

The best performing teams and team members have the appropriate numbers of members with the skills to achieve the task. More complex tasks, such as healthcare, require teams with a diverse range of skills.

Team-working processes

Mechanisms and processes must be in place to ensure effective collaboration and co-ordination between team members, particularly when members are from different professional groups. Developing effective team processes is probably the single most powerful element in team working that is likely to affect doctors' performance.

Are there reliable ways of measuring those aspects of teamwork that affect doctors' performance?

West and Markiewicz (2003) have developed questionnaires to assist in measuring most aspects of team performance. The performance criteria are specific to the team. The main instrument is the Team Performance Inventory (TPI). This reliable and validated measure is designed to assess the performance of teams in relation to the input-process-output model described earlier. It is also helpful in identifying causes when a team or individuals within a team are underperforming.

Others are developing ways to consider the processes and effectiveness of specific health service teams, such as anaesthetics, surgery and Accident and Emergency.

Are there reliable ways of intervening to change teamwork in order to improve a doctor's performance?

Tannenbaum, Salas and Cannon-Bowers (1996) reviewed research in this area and developed a model of team working that integrates interventions.

Team building

Parallel to the development of teams as principal functional units of organisations has come the development of myriad team-building interventions offered by consultants, popular books and personnel specialists. Recent reviews of the effectiveness of team-building interventions have shown that, while they often have a reliable effect upon team members' attitudes to and perceptions of one another, there is little impact upon team task performance.

Most team-building interventions focus on team relationships and cohesiveness, and are based on the mistaken assumption that improvements in cohesiveness lead to improvements in team task performance. In the few interventions which have focused on task issues there appears to be some improvement in task-related performance, but not consistently so. Team-building interventions focusing on task performance can be divided into different approaches:

- One of the most effective ways of intervening to promote their effective performance is to train leaders and facilitators (the latter should be team members). Eventually, such expertise can be extended to all team members (and should arguably be a part of pre-professional training).
- Another is to encourage a focus on patient views, providing the means whereby the team can listen to, share, and act upon information from patients or carers. Most mental health enquiries show that staff have not heard or sought the views of carers or other relatives who may have much greater knowledge of patients than they do (Reith, 1998).

Conclusion

There is substantial evidence about the factors that are associated with team and team member effectiveness. These include the input factors that should be taken into account when creating teams and team-based working, and the process factors that need to be in place to ensure that the contributions of individual team members are co-ordinated and integrated.

Five themes underlie this review. First, in today's dynamic healthcare organisations characterised by high demands and rapidly changing structures and cultures, we can enhance performance by team members taking time to reflect upon their functioning. This allows them to achieve better ways of meeting the needs of patients. Second, teams need to find creative ways of working which challenge existing orthodoxies and offer alternatives to the status quo. Such creativity comes from constructive conflict, and a preparedness to tolerate and even encourage uncertainty and ambiguity in teams composed of diverse healthcare professionals. Third, in demanding, changing and uncertain environments people must support one another to create climates of safety, confidence and empowerment. Fourth, organisations must provide nourishing and stimulating environments for teamwork. Fifth, effective and clear team leadership is vital if healthcare teams and all the professionals who work within them are to provide effective patient care while enhancing their own wellbeing and development.

References

Adorian D *et al.* (1990) Group discussions with the health care team – a method of improving care of hypertension in general practice. *Journal of Human Hypertension.* 4(3): 265–8.

Alexander JA *et al.* (1996) The effects of treatment team diversity and size on assessments of team functioning. *Hospital & Health Services Administration.* 41(1): 37–53.

Amabile TM (1983) The social psychology of creativity: A componential conceptualization. *Journal of Personality and Social Psychology.* 45: 357–76.

Borrill C *et al.* (2000) Team working and effectiveness in health care. *British Journal of Health Care Management.* 6: 364–71.

Borrill CS *et al.* (2001) *The Effectiveness of Health Care Teams in the National Health Service.* University of Aston, Birmingham.

Brown R (2000) *Group Processes* (2e). Blackwell, Oxford.

Campion MA, Medsker GJ and Higgs AC (1993) Relations between work group characteristics and effectiveness: Implications for designing effective work groups. *Personnel Psychology.* 46: 823–50.

Carter AJ and West MA (1999) Sharing the burden: team work in health care setting. In: J Firth-Cozens and R Payne (eds) *Stress in Health Professionals: psychological and organisational causes and interventions.* John Wiley & Sons, Chichester, pp. 191–202.

DeDreu CKW (1997) Productive conflict: the importance of conflict management and conflict issues. In: CKW DeDreu and E Van De Vliert (eds) *Using Conflict in Organisations.* Sage, London, pp. 9–22.

DeDreu CKW and De Vries NK (1997) Minority dissent in organisations. In: CKW DeDreu and E Van De Vliert (eds) *Using Conflict in Organisations.* Sage, London, pp. 72–86.

DeDreu CKW and De Vries NK (1993) Numerical support, information processing, and attitude change. *European Journal of Social Psychology.* 23: 647–62.

DeDreu CKW and Weingart LR (2003) Task versus relationship conflict, team performance, and team member satisfaction: A meta-analysis. *Journal of Applied Psychology.* 88(4): 741–9.

Department of Health Expert Group (2000) *An Organisation with a Memory: report of an expert group on learning from adverse events in the NHS chaired by the Chief Medical Officer* [online]. Stationery Office, London. Available at: www.dh.gov.uk/assetRoot/04/06/50/86/04065086.pdf [Accessed 15 October 2004].

Drory A and Shamir B (1988) Effects of organisational and life variables on job satisfaction and burnout. *Group and Organisation Studies.* 13(4): 441–55.

Dunbar K (1997) How scientists think: On-line creativity and conceptual change in science. In: TB Ward, SM Smith and J Vaid (eds) *Creative Thought: an investigation of conceptual structures and processes.* American Psychological Association, Washington, DC, pp. 461–93.

Eagly AH and Johnson BT (1990) Leader and leadership style: A meta-analysis. *Journal of Applied Psychology.* 108: 233–56.

Edmondson AC (1996) Learning from mistakes is easier said than done: Group and organizational influences on the detection and correction of human error. *Journal of Applied Behavioral Science.* 32(1): 5–28.

Edmondson AC (1999) Psychological safety and learning behaviour in work teams. *Administrative Science Quarterly.* 44: 350–83.

Firth-Cozens J (2001) Teams, Culture and Managing Risk. In: C Vincent (ed.) *Clinical Risk Management* (2e). BMJ Books, London.

Firth-Cozens J (2004) Organisational trust: the keystone to patient safety. *Quality & Safety in Health Care.* 13: 56–61.

Firth-Cozens J (1998) Celebrating teamwork. *Quality in Health Care.* 7(Suppl): S3–S7.

Foushee HC and Helmreich RL (1988) Group interaction and flight crew performance. In: EL Wiener and DC Nagel (eds) *Human Factors in Aviation.* Academic Press, San Diego, CA, pp. 189–227.

Guzzo RA and Dickson MW (1996) Teams in organisations: Recent research on performance and effectiveness. *Annual Review of Psychology.* **46**: 307–38.

Hackman JR (1990) *Groups That Work (And Those That Don't).* Jossey Bass, San Francisco.

Hackman JR (1992) Group influences on individuals in organisations. In: MD Dunnette and LM Hough (eds) *Handbook of Industrial and Organisational Psychology.* **3**: 199–267. Consulting Psychologists Press, Palo Alto, CA.

Hackman JR (2002) *Leading Teams: Setting the stage for great performances.* Harvard Business School, Harvard, MA.

Hackman JR and Lawler EE (1971) Employee reactions to job characteristics. *Journal of Applied Psychology.* **55**: 259–86.

Hackman JR and Oldham G (1975) Development of the job diagnostic survey. *Journal of Applied Psychology.* **60**: 159–70.

Hogg M and Abrams D (1988) *Social Identifications: a social psychology of intergroup relations and group processes.* Routledge, London.

Houston DM and Allt SK (1997) Psychological distress and error making among junior house officers. *British Journal of Health Psychology.* **12**(2): 141–51.

Hughes SL *et al.* (1992) A randomized trial of the cost effectiveness of VA hospital-based home care for the terminally ill. *Health Services Research.* **26**(6): 801–17.

Jackson SE (1996) The consequences of diversity in multidisciplinary work teams. In: MA West (ed.) *Handbook of Work Group Psychology.* John Wiley & Sons, Chichester, pp. 53–75.

Jackson G *et al.* (1993) A new community mental health team based in primary care. A description of the service and its effect on service use in the first year. *British Journal of Psychiatry.* **162**: 375–84.

Jansson A, Isacsson A and Lindholm LH (1992) Organization of health care teams and the population's contacts with primary care. *Scandinavian Journal of Primary Health Care.* **10**(4): 257–65.

Jenkins VA, Fallowfield LJ and Poole K (2001) Are members of multidisciplinary teams in breast cancer aware of each other's informational roles? *Quality in Health Care.* **10**: 70–5.

Jones RVH (1992) Teamworking in primary care: how do we know about it? *Journal of Interprofessional Care.* **6**: 25–9.

Jussim L (1986) Self-fulfilling prophecies: A theoretical and integrative review. *Psychological Review.* **93**(1): 429–45.

Jussim L, Coleman LM and Lerch (1987) The nature of stereotypes: A comparison and integration of 3 theories. *Journal of Personality and Social Psychology.* **52**(3): 536–46.

Kanter RM (1983) *The Change Masters: Corporate entrepreneurs at work.* Simon & Schuster, New York.

Kimble CE, Marsh NB and Kiska AC (1984) Sex, age and cultural differences in self-reported assertiveness. *Psychological Reports.* **55**: 419–22.

Kivimaki M, Sutinen R, Elovainion M, Vahtera J, Rasanen K, Toyry S, Ferrie JE and Firth-Cozens J (2001) Sickness absence in hospital physicians: 2 year follow-up study on determinants. *Occup & Environ Medicine.* **58**: 361–6.

LaFrance M and Mayo C (1978) *Moving Bodies: nonverbal communication in social relationships.* Brooks/Cole, Monterey, CA.

Locke E and Latham G (1991) *A Theory of Goal Setting and Task Motivation.* Prentice-Hall, Englewood Cliffs, NJ.

Luce A, Firth-Cozens J, van Zwanenberg T, Newton J *et al.* (2002) *Predicting Early Retirement in General Practice: relationship of retirement to job factors, stress and quality.* Report to NHS Executive Northern & Yorkshire.

Mathieu JE, Marks MA and Zaccaro SJ (2001) Multiteam systems. In: N Anderson, DS Ones, HK Sinangil and C Viswesvaran (eds) *Handbook of Industrial, Work and Organizational Psychology.* **2**: 289–313. Sage, London.

Mathison DL and Tucker RK (1982) Sex differences in assertive behaviour: a research extension. *Psychological Reports.* **51**(3): 943–8.

Milliken FJ and Martins LL (1996) Searching for common threads: understanding the multiple effects of diversity in organizational groups. *Academy of Management Review.* **21**(2): 402–33.

Mumford MD and Gustafson SB (1988) Creativity syndrome: integration, application and innovation. *Psychological Bulletin.* **103**: 27–43.

Nemeth CJ and Nemeth Brown B (2003) Better than individuals? The potential benefits of dissent and diversity for group creativity. In: PB Paulus and BJ Nijstad (eds) *Group Creativity: innovation through collaboration.* Oxford University Press, Oxford, pp. 63–84.

Nemeth C and Owens P (1996) Making work groups more effective: The value of minority dissent. In: MA West (ed.) *Handbook of Work Group Psychology.* John Wiley & Sons, Chichester, pp. 125–42.

Newton J, Luce A, van Zwanenberg T and Firth-Cozens J (2004) Job dissatisfaction and early retirement: a qualitative study of general practitioners in the Northern Deanery. *Primary Health Care Research and Development.* **5**(1): 68–76.

Nievaard AC (1987) Communication climate and patient care: causes and effects of nurses' attitudes to patients. *Social Science and Medicine.* **24**(9): 777–84.

Paulus PB and Nijstad BA (eds) (2003) *Group Creativity: innovation through collaboration.* Oxford University Press, Oxford.

Reith M (1998) Risk assessment and management: lessons from mental health inquiry reports. *Medical Science Law.* **38**(3): 221–6.

Roethlisberger FJ and Dixon WJ (1939) *Management and the Worker.* Harvard University Press, Cambridge, MA.

Ross F, Rink E and Furne A (2000) Integration or pragmatic coalition? An evaluation of nursing teams in primary care. *Journal of Interprofessional Care.* **14**(3): 259–67.

Sommers LS *et al.* (2000) Physician, nurse and social worker collaboration in primary care for chronically ill seniors. *Archives of Internal Medicine.* **160**(12): 1825–33.

Tajfel H (1978) The psychological structure of intergroup relations. In: H Tajfel (ed.) *Differentiation Between Social Groups: studies in the social psychology of intergroup relations.* Academic Press, London.

Tajfel H and Turner JC (1979) An integrative theory on intergroup conflict. In: WG Austin and S Worchel (eds) *The Social Psychology of Intergroup Relations.* Brooks-Cole, Monterey, CA.

Tannenbaum SI, Salas E and Cannon-Bowers JA (1996) Promoting team effectiveness. In: MA West (ed.) *Handbook of Work Group Psychology.* John Wiley & Sons, Chichester, pp. 503–29.

Tjosvold D (1991) *Team Organisation: an enduring competitive advantage.* John Wiley & Sons, Chichester.

Tjosvold D (1998) Co-operative and competitive goal approaches to conflict: accomplishments and challenges. *Applied Psychology: An International Review.* **41**: 285–342.

Wall TD *et al.* (1997) Minor psychiatric disorder in NHS trust staff: occupational and gender differences. *British Journal of Psychiatry.* **171**: 519–23.

Watson WE, Kumar K and Michaelsen LK (1993) Cultural diversity's impact on interaction process and performance: Comparing homogeneous and diverse task groups. *Academy of Management Journal.* **36**: 590–602.

West MA (1990) The social psychology of innovation in groups. In: MA West and JL Farr (eds) *Innovation and Creativity at Work: psychological and organisational strategies.* John Wiley & Sons, Chichester, pp. 309–33.

West MA (2000) Reflexivity, revolution and innovation in work teams. In: M Beyerlein (ed.) *Product Development Teams: advances in interdisciplinary studies of work teams.* JAI Press, California, pp. 1–30.

West MA and Anderson N (1996) Innovation in top management teams. *Journal of Applied Psychology.* **81**(6): 680–93.

West MA, Borrill CS and Unsworth KL (1998) Team Effectiveness in Organisations. *International Review of Industrial and Organisational Psychology.* **13**: 1–48.

West M and Field D (1995) Teamwork in primary health care. Perspectives from organisational psychology. *Journal of Interprofessional Care.* **9**: 117–22.

West MA and Markiewicz L (2003) *Building Team-Based Working: a practical guide to organizational transformation.* Blackwell Publishing Inc, Malden, USA.

West MA, Patterson MG and Dawson J (1999) A path to profit? Teamwork at the top. *Centre Piece: the Magazine of Economic Performance.* **4**(3): 7–11.

West MA and Poulton BC (1995) *Primary Health Care Teams: rhetoric versus reality.* Paper submitted for publication. Institute of Work Psychology, University of Sheffield.

West MA, Tjosvold D and Smith KG (eds) (2003) *International Handbook of Organisational Teamwork and Cooperative Working.* John Wiley & Sons, Chichester.

West MA and Wallace M (1991) Innovation in health care teams. *European Journal of Social Psychology.* **21**(4): 303–15.

West MA *et al.* (2002) The link between management of employees and patient mortality in acute hospitals. *International Journal of Human Resource Management.* **13**(8): 1299–310.

West MA *et al.* (2003) *The Relationship between Staff Management Practices and Patient Mortality in Acute Hospitals: a longitudinal study.* Aston Business School Working Paper Series, Birmingham.

Wood N, Farrow S and Elliott B (1994) A review of primary health-care organization. *Journal of Clinical Nursing.* **3**(4): 243–50.

Yeatts DE and Seward RR (2000) Reducing turnover and improving health care in nursing homes: the potential effects of self-managed work teams. *Gerontologist.* **40**(3): 358–63.

Chapter 9

Leadership and the quality of healthcare*

Jenny Firth-Cozens

Good leadership is acknowledged as essential for any type of organisation, from government to football teams and global enterprises. Recognition of its key role within healthcare has had a rather slower development than in industry, but has now been acknowledged as vital (Department of Health, 1999), particularly in the development of quality care through clinical governance. Leadership of hospital trust and management boards, for example, has been shown to be one of the most common features that distinguish between success or failure to deliver high-quality services in the NHS. However, rhetoric does not ensure good care, and so this chapter looks at the evidence for why leadership matters, what various theories of leadership tell us, what makes a leader trustworthy, and what the implications of this are for health policy, quality and leadership development in the NHS. Inevitably, the paper overlaps with teamwork, organisational culture, personality and behaviour. Finally, consideration is given to the influence of leadership on the performance of individual clinicians.

Who is leader?

Leadership exists at every level throughout an organisation (Ilgen, 1999). In healthcare it runs from government ministers through health authorities and other agencies to Trust chief executives and their Boards. It exists at almost all levels throughout their organisations, including service and professional groups, wards and primary care practices. For the patient, leadership is rarely seen; at most it may be apparent at the level of the multidisciplinary team, usually in the form of the consultant or general practitioner.

There is often a distinction made between leadership and management (Kotter, 1990). Management is usually seen as the seeking of order and stability, while leadership is more often about seeking adaptive and constructive change. At every level of an organisation both leadership and management are necessary, though in varying proportions. Leaders are likely to want to be able to produce and manage periods of stability, often at the same time as planning future changes. For this reason the two inevitably overlap, and the later discussion of transformational and transactional leadership styles reflects this.

---

* This review is based on a number of papers: Firth-Cozens and Mowbray (2001) Leadership and the quality of care. *Quality in Health Care.* 10(suppl II): ii3–ii7; Firth-Cozens (2001) Cultures for improving patient safety through learning: the role of teamwork. *Quality in Health Care.* 10(suppl II): ii, 0–6, and Firth-Cozens. Organisational trust: the keystone to patient safety. *Quality & Safety in Health Care* (in press).

It has probably been unhelpful to distinguish management and leadership to the extent that this has happened in recent years – it can encourage chief executives to think of leadership as purely a driving of the new, leaving others to implement and maintain systems. This may not be useful or appropriate.

Leadership research

Leadership research is wide-ranging, covering the different values and abilities which make up the concept itself: the leader's personality or behaviour; the people who are led (including their culture); and the context, such as the type of organisation (for example, healthcare or car production), as well as the wider context faced by that organisation at the time. Through the combination of these we can begin to appreciate the true complexity of what it means to lead any particular group of people successfully. Advances in leadership theory involve a consideration of the leader's characteristics, behaviours and the situation simultaneously (Sashkin, 1989). Much leadership research is contained within studies of organisational culture and teamwork (*see* Chapters 7 and 8). Within healthcare, useful research on leadership also links these factors to quality, patient safety and efficiency.

The variables which have been shown to be positive or negative for leadership are outlined in the following sections and summarised in Table 9.1.

Table 9.1 Positive and negative leadership attributes

Positive Attributes	Negative Attributes
Intelligent*	[The opposite of those in column 1]
Has ability*	Dictatorial/authoritarian**
Confident**	Arrogant
Warm and friendly**	Hostile
Benevolent*	Boastful/promotes own ideas
Emotionally stable*	Laissez-faire
Able to recognise limitations	
Has integrity*	
Able to delegate/share load*	
Skills:	
Good communication skills*	
Creates a sense of justice	
Gives staff control and discretion	
Can anticipate events and plan to address them	

* At least two references to this attribute. ** At least three references to this attribute.

The personalities of good leaders

Some leaders emerge because of their own influence and the support of others, including staff. Others are given their roles. Emergent leaders in a student population have been shown to be more dominant, intelligent and confident about their own performance and identified more often as leaders by others in the group (Smith & Foti, 1998). Some are short-term leaders, useful in producing short-term goals, but who do not manage longer-term ones which involve carrying their staff with them. Such findings on student groups show some commonality with studies which look at performance and outcomes emerging from different types of personality and leadership characteristics.

For example, research with airline crews found that error levels were lowest where the leaders were warm, friendly, self-confident and able to stand up to pressure and highest when they were arrogant, hostile, boastful or dictatorial (Chidester *et al.*, 1991). These traits relate to 'Agreeableness' and 'Emotional Stability' (Hogan, Curphy & Hogan, 1994), two of the so-called Big Five personality constructs which are used for job selection. These are discussed in more detail in Chapter 5. Other studies which have looked at 'great leaders' – such as Churchill, Alexander the Great, Henry V or famous business leaders – come up with a similar collection of characteristics including intelligence, self-confidence, determination, integrity and sociability (Northouse, 2001).

Within health services 'opinion leaders' are also seen as important – for example, clinicians who have been shown to be influential in introducing evidence-based healthcare (Thomson O'Brien *et al.*, 2001). They provide strong role models for the beliefs and values they wish others to adopt, appear competent to those they lead, and are able to articulate ideological goals (House, 1977). Within a clinical setting such leadership skills are very valuable as long as they are in line with the aims of the organisation as a whole; that is, to provide effective, quality care. If their goals are in another direction, leaders can lead their teams or staff astray. This is particularly important in self-managed teams (Firth-Cozens, 2001b).

These findings coincide with the 'man-on-the-street's' picture of the strong, extravert, confident leader, and may also be what patients want to see in their clinicians. However, staff may want different types of leaders to those seen as best by customers or patients. A UK study, where NHS staff and leaders were asked what they considered made a good leader, concluded that staff wanted leaders who could do the best for them – what they called 'the model of leader as servant' (Alimo-Metcalfe & Alban-Metcalfe, 2000). It may be that, in organisations where staff have to give so much to others, they need a more caring, benevolent type of leadership. Although the fact that staff want this type of leader has not been linked to outcomes, as described later, what is best for staff appears to be best for patients too.

Trustworthy leaders

After a series of alarming audits of healthcare accidents in the US, UK and Australia, healthcare is modelling itself to some extent upon the aviation industry, which has used reporting and learning from error as a means to increase its safety record (Department of Health Expert Group, 2000; Helmreich, 2000). However, reporting errors – whether one's own or those of a colleague – is not something which comes easily to NHS staff (Vincent, Stanhope & Crowley-Murphy, 1999). Barriers to such reporting include poor leadership and a culture of fear (Firth-Cozens, 2003).

The links between error-reporting, team functioning and leadership have been demonstrated by Edmondson (Edmondson, 1996), who showed that the personality of the leader played a part in the number of errors recorded. Looking at the relationship between medication errors and the quality of nursing teamwork, she found that good teams recorded more errors than poor teams. To explore this further she interviewed the team leaders themselves, and found that authoritarian, dictatorial leaders led the poorer teams, who reported, perhaps not surprisingly, fewer errors.

This shows how carefully healthcare data should be interpreted: if a regime is repressive or dictatorial, its staff are almost bound to produce data which are less than accurate. Leaders should perhaps be judged more by demonstrating how good their teams are at detecting errors and problems and learning from them, and less by the number of errors reported. This might also be an indication of how trustworthy the leader is perceived to be by staff.

A number of studies have looked at what makes up a trustworthy leader and found that this concept comes from three principal characteristics: their ability, their benevolence and their integrity (Mayer, Davis & Schoorman, 1995).

Ability is an amalgamation of skills and competencies, including being able to influence others. For most people, ability is limited to a single domain, such as clinical work or financial management, although trusting someone's ability in less concrete skills may cover a number of domains. These underlying qualities of leadership include being able to set direction, work collaboratively, be empowering and politically astute, be able to select good staff, and generally to deliver the service needed. (A framework of the abilities required by NHS leaders is set out in www.nhsleadershipqualities.nhs.uk.)

Benevolence, or the demonstration of concern, is a particularly important characteristic in terms of the trust needed to ensure good quality care. Research has shown NHS staff want 'the model of leader as servant' (Alimo-Metcalfe & Alban-Metcalfe, 2000) – as described above. They need the leader to be seen to be on their side, to be able to understand their problems and be benevolent if things go wrong.

Leaders need to be able to demonstrate that they understand the difficulties faced by staff, value their staff and have positive intentions towards them and to their patients: a leader is more likely to be seen as understanding and benevolent if he or she is seen regularly at the coal face, experiencing fully the difficulties and anxieties of staff and patients (Schellekens & Bisognano, 2001), valuing good work done and consulting with staff on ways to make it better.

Integrity is the third characteristic of trustworthy leadership. Leaders must demonstrate their values and principles; for example, keeping their word that adverse events will be treated non-punitively so long as staff adhere to safety protocols or agreed responsibilities. An expedient leader who tolerates poor quality may lose trust. Demonstrating integrity can be a real challenge to leaders if they are given conflicting roles by government – to show greater and greater efficiency while at the same time increasing the quality of care, or to gather information for the purpose of learning about safety whilst dealing benevolently or fairly with cases which hit the media. Unless integrity, benevolence and competence are shown to healthcare leaders by those who control *them*, they are going to find it particularly difficult to have the strength to treat their staff in ways which will increase their trust.

Leadership and decision making

Different leadership types affect decisions reached. One study tested the ways leaders affected the level of 'groupthink' in a team (Ahlfinger & Esser, 2001). Groupthink occurs where teams close up against outside messages or even from isolated individuals within the team (for example, ING Barings collapse), and strive prematurely for unanimous agreement on a course of action (Janis, 1982; Roberts & Bea, 2001). Groups with 'promotional leaders' – ones who promote their own preferred solutions – produce more groupthink, discuss fewer facts, and reach decisions more quickly than groups with non-promotional leaders (Ahlfinger & Esser, 2001). This has important implications for both clinical and management teams in healthcare where multidisciplinary teamwork and decision making are so important.

Type and leadership

Different ways of leading have implications for those around and potentially for healthcare. The Myers Briggs Type Indicator (MBTI) (Kirby, 1997; Kroeger & Thuesen, 1993) described in Chapter 5, does not describe the characteristics of the best leaders. Rather it celebrates difference, saying that a person with any group of characteristics and preferences which make up one of 16 personality types can lead as well as any other, but is likely to lead differently. (For a popular but good account of type theory see Kroeger & Thuesen (1993).) The four dimensions of the MBTI are also described in Chapter 5.

Good leadership for an organisation is likely to need aspects of both parts of each MBTI personality dimension. For example, leaders have sometimes to make decisions which are logical, but they also need to be aware of the effects this might have on people. 'Sensing' leaders might adhere to detail in the present and be able to use the past well, but it is also vital to be able to plan for the future, anticipate safety and quality and other problems and solve them before they happen – something that might come more naturally to those with a more intuitive preference.

A principal attribute for good leaders is to recognise the strengths and weaknesses that result from their particular personality type, to develop their 'least preferred areas' and to recognise and reward the different skills of others in the team or in different sections of the organisation (Clack et al., 2004).

Because of career preferences, there is inevitably a preponderance of a particular type in different sections of an organisation. For example, chief executives are likely to be predominantly extrovert, and consultants mainly introvert (Walck, 1997; Clack et al., 2004), while nurses mainly make decisions according to value systems concerning people rather than the sense of what is logical and rational – an approach which may be preferred by their doctor and manager colleagues. For example, a senior doctor in difficulties who was value-driven and found himself in trouble for standing up for patients against other doctors on more than one occasion would rather spend time with nurses than with medical colleagues. This did not help his reputation. Explaining the differences between the MBTI 'Feelings' type and the 'Thinking' type and the likely differences between him and his colleagues gave him insight into his difficulties and he learnt ways to communicate and act with 'Thinking' types while still holding his own values. Such differences in type affect communication, persuasion and decision making and can lead to accusations of bullying.

Type theory is therefore invaluable for understanding why a particular doctor is having interpersonal problems in a team or with management or patients. This applies, whether the person is a leader or having difficulties with his or her leader.

Leadership styles and quality

One of the most enduring distinctions in leadership research is between the two styles of transactional and transformational leadership.

Transactional leadership stems from a traditional view of the leader having power and authority over followers, and the use of power to achieve goals and objectives (Burns, 1979).

The principal components of this leadership style are contingent rewards for staff, and management by exception, which involves a focus on problems and mistakes. Some might say that the UK government's management of the health service fits this mode of leadership and that the style flows down to most healthcare organisations and even clinical teams. It may be less common in primary care.

Transformational leadership looks for ways to motivate followers with a view to engaging them more intimately in the process of work; it is 'performance beyond expectations' (Bass, 1985). Transformational leaders can initiate and cope with change, and create something new from something old. They are entrepreneurial, take and anticipate risks, and are often informal in their relationships, always seeking to develop individuals and respond to their needs and interests.

Researchers found that NHS staff needed both transformational and transactional leadership. Research has failed to show conclusively that transformational leaders are always best (Masi & Cooke, 2000). The model of the transformational leader creating rapid change (seen in the NHS over the past 15 years) is not always beneficial for the remaining staff, nor for the rounded development of the leader, and so probably not for patients either. Leaders should recognise their own style and work as much as possible with those with complementary styles.

Teams, leaders and quality

There are theoretical and commonsense reasons why and how leaders might affect the final product that is delivered by their organisations or their teams; in this case, patient care. There is also a small but growing area of research which confirms some of these reasons and provides evidence for a pathway of care from the leader through the staff to the patients themselves.

The relationships between these factors are shown in Figure 9.1. Working back from the professional–patient interface, there is evidence that stressed staff produce inferior care (Firth-Cozens, 2001a). Evidence has come, for example, from cognitive testing, looking at the effects of fatigue on decision making (Smith, 2001) and looking at the relationships between stress, insomnia and errors and how the relationship strengthens over time as junior doctors begin new posts (Houston & Allt, 1997).

Stress in health service staff, at least in the National Health Service, is considerably higher than in other members of the workforce, with around 28% showing

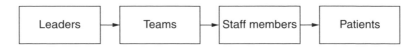

Figure 9.1 Links between outside forces, leaders, teams, staff and patient care.

levels above threshold for symptoms. In one study of the effects of work stress on patient care, young doctors described events from general carelessness through to errors contributing to patient deaths which they attributed primarily to their exhaustion, overwork, lack of support or the symptoms of depression (Firth-Cozens & Greenhalgh, 1997). Forty per cent of the doctors described became irritable or even abusive to patients and colleagues, showing the effects on patient care and around the team itself. The largest patient satisfaction survey ever conducted showed that the highest correlations were with the cheerfulness, friendliness and sensitivity of staff (Press Ganey Associates, 1997). Clearly the psychological well-being of staff affects the quality of patient care in a variety of ways.

Clearly tackling job stress is a crucial step in producing better care. There is growing evidence that team functioning is an important predictor of stress levels (Firth-Cozens & Rayner, 2000; Carter & West, 1999). In a study of NHS health staff in 19 organisations, those who reported being in no teams had the highest stress levels, followed by those in teams with inferior functioning, with those in well-functioning teams having the fewest symptoms (Carter & West, 1999). Members of a well-functioning team are able to provide support to each other and step in to help when necessary (Firth-Cozens, 2001b; Morgan et al., 1986). The relationship between teamwork and performance is covered in more detail in Chapter 8.

Both team and individual functioning are affected by leaders, and meta-analytic studies have shown that the principal cause of workplace stress is 'the boss' (Hogan, Raskin & Fazzini, 1990), and so it is reasonable to suppose that good leadership produces good teams with low stress and better patient care. One way that this might happen is through the perceptiveness of the leader to the needs and views of their staff. In a recent study (Firth-Cozens & Rayner, 2000) we compared house officers' attitudes to work and stress levels with their consultants' views of their house officers' attitudes to work. The 'gap' between the consultants' views and their house officers' views was highly related to staff stress levels. The 'gap' was a large predictor of whether the team was functioning well or not. In other words, the team leader's skills in accurately recognising the views of his or her staff members was an extremely important factor in the latter's stress levels and in the quality of team-work. These studies show a clear path back through patient care to staff stress to team leadership.

Another way that leaders may influence quality of care is in their attitudes to safety which, in other industries, have been shown to be reflected by their staff and related to the number of accidents (O'Toole, 2002). Leaders influence both the organisational culture (in terms of safety) but also actual performance; for example, by recognition of their 'sapiential authority' – which comes from experience and being on hand in an emergency, etc. – rather than their formal status (Boreham, Shea & Mackway-Jones, 2000). Similarly, ability to appreciate one's limits and use the crew/team widely and wisely are important attributes of excellent pilots (Helmreich et al., 1986).

Corrigan et al. (2000) measured leadership style in 31 mental health teams and asked their clients to rate their satisfaction with the treatment programmes and their quality of life. Both factors were inversely associated with laissez-faire leadership styles and positively associated with both transformational and transactional leadership. The leaders' and subordinates' ratings of their team leadership independently accounted for 40% of the total variance in client satisfaction.

Other evidence of the effects of leaders on surgical outcomes comes from the study by Carthey *et al.* (2003) of behaviours and their relationship to error and compensation. The behavioural markers for good outcomes in surgeons were factors such as clear communication style, high safety awareness, cognitive flexibility and mental resilience. The numbers in this study were small, but the use of behavioural markers is probably more accurate than looking at attitudes or personality as reported by the individual. Nevertheless, leadership style in terms of personality and attitudes determined from psychometric questionnaires does affect safety, as we saw above with research with airline pilots (Chidester *et al.*, 1991; Helmreich *et al.*, 1986) and with differences in accurately reporting error (Edmondson, 1996).

This section has shown that leaders affect patient care and satisfaction through their management of teams and the effects this has on the stress levels of their team members, including doctors. Although most evidence comes from teams, it is likely that this is also true for the effect of chief executives on whole organisations. It implies again that as well as assessing leaders by their meeting assigned objectives, their effectiveness should be assessed by the stress levels or wellbeing – absence, turnover, disruptive behaviours (Townsend, Phillipps & Elkins, 2000) – of their staff. We also need to remember that the context in which leaders operate affects their ability to lead well or not.

Is NHS leadership different?

As in other industries, transformational leadership continues to be the style that is presumed best for health services, primarily because it has a focus on change. However, it is not always easy to achieve because most change is imposed upon NHS leaders and its expected outcomes are detailed. Transactional methods of performance monitoring: clinical audit, re-accreditation, controls assurance, central error reporting, league tables, etc., which are all laudable in their intention and valuable in themselves, influence leaders to take a more transactional style than they might otherwise have done. The more centralised such controls become, the less a leader is able to give staff the discretion and participation which they desire (Alimo-Metcalfe & Alban-Metcalfe, 2000; Firth-Cozens, in press). The first and central conflict in the NHS agenda for better health services is to make staff accountable while allowing their creativity and participation to flourish. As such it poses a major challenge for the leaders of that agenda.

A second conflict for health service leaders is between quality and efficiency which may affect the consistency of behaviour and integrity necessary for the development of trust. This is not always easy in the NHS. The reality for healthcare leaders is often one of desperate choices which affect consistency and the provision of quality care. For example, an inner city general practitioner may be in vital need of a partner, but have no other option than a known but not entirely trusted locum (West, 2001).

The third conflict is that NHS leadership, through its directors and chief executives, differs from other leadership settings in a fundamental way. Despite the great achievement of the NHS in treating one million patients a day, there is always the presence of a dark side – disease, distress, disability and death. Because of this there is a natural tendency for non-clinical leaders to fail to appreciate what is happening on the front line in ways which are much less applicable to other industries. Leaders in the health service have to face the fact that staff doing their best is often not enough: mistakes and poor care happen, and people – staff and patients alike – can suffer badly as a result. Leaders must be emotionally strong enough to get close to patients' and staff's experiences – to do what has been called 'the walk of shame' (Schellekens & Bisognano, 2001) – but they need training and support for this.

These difficulties in NHS leadership are different to those elsewhere. Leadership training and development must take them into account and help people to tackle them rather than using models from less complex cultures.

It is possible for some leaders to achieve targets and objectives successfully and quickly, but at the cost of a demoralised and highly stressed workforce. If these leaders move swiftly onwards and upwards as a result of their more obvious achievements, the organisation is likely to suffer and perform less well in the subsequent period.

Assessment of leadership

Apart from measuring achievement of objectives, assessment of leadership can be done in a variety of ways. One is to measure staff stress levels.

Successful leaders have staff with relatively low stress levels and who report errors and problems in their work as easily as they report successes. This indicates a reasonably safety-conscious and supportive organisational culture. A staff survey, using the 12-item General Health Questionnaire, will be a good indicator of stress levels. Based upon previous surveys in healthcare organisations (*see* Chapter 5), it would be reasonable to consider that those organisations or departments with at least 80% below the threshold score of 4 were doing reasonably well, while those with less than 70% below threshold were those giving cause for concern, unless there were good contextual reasons for this, such as difficult organisational change.

Trustworthiness can be tested objectively by the way poor performance and problems are reported without comeback, and solutions and improvements brought about as a result. Leaders can be assessed by using 360-degree feedback over two well-spaced assessments: most people will have some negative feedback, so an ability to improve should be an important consideration.

Good appraisal processes are also useful, particularly in developing leadership qualities. A gaining of self-awareness through coaching and mentoring should also be seen as an achievement. Healthcare leaders require support in facing difficult conflicts concerning their integrity and the difficult roles faced by their staff. Such support should come through good mentoring, as well as through support from their superiors in difficult times as well as good ones.

Conclusion

This chapter argues that good leadership benefits patient care and describes some of the behaviours and characteristics that underpin it. These are summarised in Table 9.1. Certain traits such as arrogance, authoritarianism and strong competitiveness may be prejudicial to good leadership, and sociable, confident people who work well under stress have a head start in making good leaders. Both transformational or transactional leadership styles are necessary for health services, and this also concurs with personality type theory (Myers Briggs). Where leaders feel more in tune with one approach than the other it may be more important to ensure that others play the role that they find more difficult rather than try to do both themselves.

References

Ahlfinger NR and Esser JK (2001) Testing the groupthink model: effects of promotional leadership and conformity predisposition. *Social Behaviour and Personality*. **29**(1): 31–42.

Alimo-Metcalfe B and Alban-Metcalfe R (2000) Leadership. Heaven can wait. *Health Service Journal*. **110**(5726): 26–9.

Bass BM (1985) *Leadership and Performance Beyond Expectations*. Harper & Row, New York.

Boreham NC, Shea CE and Mackway-Jones K (2000) Clinical risk and collective competence in the hospital emergency department in the UK. *Social Science and Medicine*. **51**(1): 83–91.

Burns JM (1979) *Leadership*. Harper Colophon, New York.

Carter AJ and West MA (1999) Sharing the burden: team work in health care setting. In: J Firth-Cozens and RL Payne (eds) *Stress in Health Professionals: psychological and organisational causes and interventions*. John Wiley & Sons, Chichester, pp. 191–202.

Carthey J *et al.* (2003) Behavioural markers of surgical excellence. *Safety Science*. **41**(5): 409–25.

Chidester TR *et al.* (1991) Pilot personality and crew coordination. *International Journal of Aviation Psychology*. **1**(1): 25–44.

Clack GB *et al.* (2004) Personality differences between doctors and their patients: implications for the teaching of communication skills. *Medical Education*. **38**(2): 177–86.

Corrigan PW *et al.* (2000) Mental health team leadership and consumers' satisfaction and quality of life. *Psychiatric Services*. **51**(6): 781–5.

Department of Health (1999) *Leadership for Health: the health authority role*. Department of Health, London.

Department of Health Expert Group (2000) *An Organisation with a Memory: report of the expert group on learning from adverse events in the NHS*. Department of Health, London.

Edmondson AC (1996) Learning from mistakes is easier said than done: group and organisational influences on the detection and correction of human error. *Journal of Applied Behavioral Science*. **32**(1): 5–28.

Firth-Cozens J (2001a) Interventions to improve physicians' well-being and patient care. *Social Science & Medicine*. **52**(2): 215–22.

Firth-Cozens J (2001b) Teams, culture and managing risk. In: C Vincent (ed.) *Clinical Risk Management* (2e). BMJ Books, London, pp. 355–68.

Firth-Cozens J (2003) Learning from error. In: J Harrison, R Innes and T van Zwanenberg (eds) *Regaining Trust in Healthcare*. Radcliffe Medical Press, Oxford.

Firth-Cozens J (2005) Managing change in mental health services. In: A James, A Worrall and T Kendall (eds) *Clinical Governance in Mental Health and Learning Disability Services: a practical guide*. Gaskell, London.

Firth-Cozens J and Greenhalgh J (1997) Doctors' perceptions of the links between stress and lowered clinical care. *Social Science and Medicine*. **44**(7): 1017–22.

Firth-Cozens J and Rayner K (2000) *Report on the Training Experiences of Pre-registration House Officers and Comparing Two Systems*. University of Northumbria at Newcastle, Newcastle upon Tyne.

Helmreich RL (2000) On error management: lessons from aviation. *BMJ*. **320**(7237): 781–5.

Helmreich RL *et al.* (1986) Cockpit resource management: exploring the attitude-performance linkage. *Aviation, Space, and Environmental Medicine*. **57**(12 part 1): 1198–200.

Hogan R, Curphy GJ and Hogan J (1994) What we know about leadership. Effectiveness and personality. *American Psychologist*. **49**(6): 493–504.

Hogan R, Raskin R and Fazzini D (1990) The dark side of charisma. In: KE Clark and MB Clark (eds) *Measures of Leadership*. Leadership Library of America, West Orange, pp. 343–54.

House RJ (1977) A theory of charismatic leadership. In: JG Hunt and LL Larson (eds) *Leadership: the cutting edge*. A Symposium held at Southern Illinois University, Carbondale, October 27–28, 1976. Southern Illinois University Press, Carbondale.

Houston DM and Allt SK (1997) Psychological distress and error making among junior house officers. *British Journal of Health Psychology*. **12**(2): 141–51.

Ilgen DR (1999) Teams embedded in organisations: Some implications. *American Psychologist*. **54**(2): 129–39.

Janis IL (1982) *Groupthink: psychological studies of policy decisions and fiascos* (2e). Houghton Mifflin, Boston.

Kirby LK (1997) Introduction: psychological type and the Myers-Briggs Type Indicator. In: C Fitzgerald and LK Kirby (eds) *Developing Leaders: research and applications in psychological type and leadership development: integrating reality and vision, mind and heart*. Davies Black Publishing, Palo Alto, CA, ch.1.

Kotter JP (1990) *A Force for Change: how leadership differs from management*. Free Press, New York.

Kroeger O and Thuesen JM (1993) *Type Talk at Work*. Delacorte Press, New York.

Masi RJ and Cooke RA (2000) Effects of transformational leadership on subordinate motivation, empowering norms and organizational productivity. *International Journal of Organizational Analysis*. **8**(1): 16–47.

Mayer RC, Davis JH and Schoorman FD (1995) An integration model of organizational trust. *Academy of Management Review*. **20**(3): 709–34.

Morgan GG Jr, Glickman AS, Woodware CA, Blaiwes A and Salas E (1986) *Measurement of Team Behaviours in a Navy Environment*. Naval Training System Center, Orlando, FL.

Northouse PG (2001) *Leadership: theory and practice* (2e). Sage Publications, London.

O'Toole M (2002) The relationship between employees' perceptions of safety and organizational culture. *Journal of Safety Research*. **33**(2): 231–43.

Press Ganey Associates (1997) *One Million Patients Have Spoken: Who will listen?* [online]. Press Ganey Associates Inc., South Bend, Indiana. Available at: www.pressganey.org/products_services/readings_findings/satmon/article.php?article_id=151 [Accessed 21 October 2004].

Roberts KH and Bea RG (2001) When systems fail. *Organizational Dynamics*. **29**(3): 179–91.

Sashkin M (1989) Visionary leadership: a perspective from education. In: WE Rosenbach and RL Taylor (eds) *Contemporary Issues in Leadership* (2e). Westview Press, Boulder, pp. 222–34.

Schellekens W and Bisognano M (2001) *Improving the Processes of Leadership*. Presented at 6th European Forum of Quality Improvement in Health Care, Bologna.

Smith JA and Foti RJ (1998) A pattern approach to the study of leader emergence. *The Leadership Quarterly*. **9**(2): 147–60.

Smith L (2001) Working time, stress and fatigue. In: C Vincent (ed.) *Clinical Risk Management*. BMJ Books, London, pp. 319–40.

Thomson O'Brien MA *et al.* (2001) Local opinion leaders: effects on professional practice and health care outcomes (Cochrane Review). In: *The Cochrane Library. Issue 4*. Update Software, Oxford.

Townsend J, Phillipps JS and Elkins TJ (2000) Employee retaliation: the neglected consequence of poor leader-member exchange relations. *Journal of Occupational Health Psychology*. **5**(4): 457–63.

Vincent C, Stanhope N and Crowley-Murphy M (1999) Reasons for not reporting adverse incidents: an empirical study. *Journal of Evaluation in Clinical Practice*. **5**(1): 13–21.

Walck CL (1997) Using the MBTI in management and leadership: a review of the literature. In: C Fitzgerald and LK Kirby (eds) *Developing Leaders: research and applications in psychological type and leadership development: integrating reality and vision, mind and heart*. Davies Black Publishing, Palo Alto, CA, ch.3.

West L (2001) *Doctors on the Edge: general practitioners, health and learning in the inner city*. Free Association Books, London.

Chapter 10

Workload, sleep loss and shift work

Lawrence Smith

Introduction

Doctors and nursing staff are well aware of the potential reduction in clinical performance as a result of sleep loss and fatigue. Despite this awareness they will sometimes be so tired that, motivationally, they will not be in an optimal state to make appropriate treatment decisions. Mistakes may be made and treatment decisions inappropriately deferred. A further aspect of long work hours, prolonged night work, workload and stress effects is the potential for interaction effects upon work performance. The end of a run of successive night duties, heavy work demands, fatigue, sleepiness, distractions in the environment and having to make crucial decisions during the circadian downturn in alertness could very well combine, irrespective of compensatory effort, to degrade clinical performance. It only takes one 'window of catastrophe' to occur in one working lifetime for the severest consequences to occur.

Medicine has become even more of a 24-hour discipline. The admission and treatment of patients routinely at night has added to overall workload. Work is more intense because of a trend towards only admitting patients to hospital with serious conditions and discharging them sooner than was once the case. This concentrates the work of medical staff who are dealing with acute and often severe problems and who may have less opportunity to relax or sleep on call and less time to interact with patients, relatives and staff. New working arrangements, including reduced working hours and shift work introduced to enable compliance with the European Working Time Directive, have both benefits and disadvantages. Whilst the reduction in the overall number of hours worked by doctors reduces some stresses, the intensity of workload, lack of continuity and need for junior doctors in particular to work as a member of a larger number of different teams are stressors in their own right. There is, to date, little research evidence on the effect of newer working practices.

What are the factors of potential influence on a doctor's performance?

The aim here is to consider three factors that have a potential influence on doctors' performance: workload, sleep loss and shift work. In particular this review is concerned with 'non-standard' working time, including shift and night work, sleep loss and workload, and their influence upon the work effectiveness and health of medical professionals. In addition, methods for assessment of factors and possible intervention strategies are suggested.

Workload

Work stress and its effects: why does the factor arise?

Workload is typically understood in terms of job demands, including the amount and type of work done and attendant time pressures. This 'real-world' view is exemplified in the few workload-related studies that have been published with regard to doctors. Workload research tends to focus on underlying cognitive processes affecting task demands, resources available and effort invested. There is a focus on 'mental workload'. This is because the successful completion of many of the primary tasks in many workplaces, including those in the health sector, involves memory, decision making, attention, perception, fine motor control and communication skills rather than substantial physical demands.

Typically, high actual and perceived workload appears to be linked to fatigue, poorer sleep and impaired performance. Experienced workload is likely to be a function of an interaction between job or task demands, strategies used to manage those demands and the adequacy of achieved task performance, rather than simply being dependent on task load. However, individual differences in responses to work schedules and workload are acknowledged.

A number of sources of stress at work have been identified, including:

- factors intrinsic to the job such as work overload/underload, time pressures, work hours, shift work, physical work conditions and repetitive work
- role-based stress such as work role ambiguity, work role conflict, and levels of responsibility (especially responsibility without control)
- conflicting demands between work and home life
- relationships/interactions with subordinates, colleagues and superiors in work and with partners/family outside work
- career development factors such as lack of job security, under-/over-promotion and thwarted ambition
- organisational structure and culture, including office politics, communications, participation in decision making, the organisation of work and organisational trust (Arnold, Cooper & Robertson, 1995).

Medical professionals also face the stresses of:

- dealing with the consequences of death and serious illness
- increasing challenges to medical decision making
- increased resort to litigation (Firth-Cozens, 1998).

Some of the effects of stress on doctors can be quite profound. For example:

- depression, linked in part to sleep loss (Firth-Cozens, 1998), and other psychiatric disorders among doctors are suggested to be relatively unacknowledged problems (Thapar, 1989)

- higher than average levels of alcoholism, drug abuse, marital breakdown and affective disorders amongst doctors (Vaillant, Sobowale & McArthur *et al.*, 1972; Murray, 1977; Firth-Cozens, 1987)
- patient care affected detrimentally, e.g. lowered standards, irritability or anger, serious mistakes and serious errors resulting in patient death (Firth-Cozens & Greenhalgh, 1997; Firth-Cozens & Morrison, 1989).

Some of the causes for these psychiatric and behavioural difficulties reported by doctors included high workload, but a link to inadequacy of sleep and rest in relation to work demands is also suggested. Stress levels have also been reported to be associated with number of hours worked (Firth-Cozens, 1995).

Workload and its effect on performance is best understood in terms of job demands and can reflect:

- the number of work tasks to attend to
- deadlines for specific tasks
- lack of control over work being done
- complexity of tasks
- risks associated with particular tasks
- psychological and/or physical orientation.

These demands are exemplified in the few workload-related studies on doctors. Workload can involve subjective stress manifested as anxiety, dissatisfaction, a sense of loss of control, decreased motivation and depleted morale – all of which have the potential to affect performance in work (Tattersall, 2000). When the strain of long work hours, shift and night work, and regular sleep loss is added to a heavy workload, the risk of reduced performance and wellbeing may be accentuated.

Tattersall (2000) notes that workload research tends to consider underlying cognitive processes in terms of:

- task demands
- resources available
- effort invested.

Much of the research focus is on 'mental workload' rather than substantial physical demands because, in many workplaces including the health sector, the successful completion of many of the primary tasks involves:

- memory
- decision making
- attention
- perception
- fine motor control
- communication skills.

Where appropriate performance is not maintained, it is worth noting that this may result from a number of factors and not workload *per se* (Tattersall, 2000).

- Effort may not be invested because motivation is low.
- Knowledge of task goals may be poor.
- Increased demands might not be attended to.
- Strategies may be used to protect resources to address future demands.

- Poor physical or emotional states caused by illness or environmental conditions might contribute to poor performance.

How does workload affect performance?

Workload does not solely rely on the task but is likely to be a function of an interaction between job demands, strategies used to manage the demands and the adequacy of task performance (Tattersall, 2000).

There may be acute and chronic implications of work demands (Tattersall, 2000). Acute effects occur where a number of tasks have to be completed at once with immediate effects on job performance. Workload may also cause problems where demands are frequent, varied and irregular or where there are short periods of intense demand interspersed by longer periods requiring little or no response.

Workload has implications for longer-term health as well as performance. The fatiguing effects of high workload (and managing it) and concurrent effects on biological and emotional states over sustained periods (overcoming fatigue is fatiguing) may lead to deterioration of job performance.

Workload and doctors

A number of studies have reported the effects of workload on the performance of doctors.

- Time pressure (an aspect of workload) and sleep loss can be major stresses for junior doctors (Ford, 1983; Hurwitz *et al.*, 1987), interfering with both learning and the provision of medical care (McCue, 1985).
- Heavy workload has been linked to chronic partial sleep deprivation. Sleep duration was negatively related to numbers of new admissions and to self-reported assessment of workload* (Tov, Rubin & Lavie, 1995).
- Unsurprisingly, hours of clinical responsibility worked have been linked to higher fatigue. Those working longer hours were more likely to register concern about heavy workloads. Stress and anxiety regarding quality of care were prevalent in junior doctors, especially where there were long hours of clinical responsibility in early training (Lewittes & Marshall, 1989).
- Relationships between sleep, perceived workload and real workload** can be inconsistent. Junior doctors respond inconsistently to on-call duty. No association was found between perceived and real workload. This was attributed to differences in doctors' working 'styles' (Tanz & Charrow, 1993).
- Doctors reported that high workload impaired ability to function efficiently (Wilkinson, Tyler & Varey, 1975).

Continued overleaf

---

* Comparisons of wards with 'light' (including oncology, dermatology, neurology, urology and radiology) and 'heavy' (mainly nights in accident and emergency) workloads have shown significant differences in doctors' sleep durations. Workload was defined as number of hospitalised patients, number of patients treated and discharged, equated for the number of doctors on duty.
** Defined in terms of: the number of admissions, number of patients, number of deaths, number of transfers and/or number of delivery room visits.

- Subjective workload has been negatively related to hours of sleep. Tendency to experience difficult on-call periods was negatively correlated with hours of sleep, but not linked to actual workload (Tanz & Charrow, 1993).
- Higher workload has been associated with sleep loss and decreased aerobic fitness (Suskin *et al.*, 1998).
- High workload was linked to burnout (emotional exhaustion and depersonalisation) and detrimental 'spill over' in terms of work-home conflicts (Geurts, Rutte & Peeters, 1999).
- Heavy workload was linked to stress, fatigue, sleep loss and effectiveness of work performance but not to clinical outcomes (Morales, Peters & Afessa, 2003).
- Level of role clarity and work-group functioning, stress and workload predict job satisfaction (Heyworth *et al.*, 1993). Interestingly, the number of hours worked did not seem to have a significant impact.

What are the existing methods for the assessment of workload and its impact on the performance of a doctor?

A number of measures have been developed to assess performance at work (O'Donnell & Eggemeier, 1986; Damos, 1991).

There are two broad approaches: primary and secondary task methods.

- The primary task is the person's work function or job.
- A secondary task method is one performed concurrently with the primary task in order to assess the workload involved with the primary task.

It can be difficult to generate a simple measure of an individual's primary task performance because people tend to invest compensatory effort when performing demanding tasks. Work demands may be underestimated because of workers' coping mechanisms. Primary task measures are most useful when performance errors or failure become apparent (Tattersall, 2000).

Secondary task measures (e.g. tests of memory, choice reaction time, time estimation and mental arithmetic) may be more sensitive to subtle changes in workload than primary task measures. Changes in performance on the secondary task reflect the performance on the primary task (e.g. Casali & Wierwille, 1983).

Subjective measures

The simplest way to measure workload is self-reporting. Self-report measures are relatively easy to use and minimally invasive and are most accurate in measuring the number of tasks or amount of work being completed (Aretz, Johannsen & Obser, 1996).

Many subjective measures of workload have been developed (see Wilson & Eggermeier, 1991, for a review), but two measures have come to prominence, namely the NASA Task Load Index (TLX: Hart & Staveland, 1988) and the Subjective Workload Assessment Technique (SWAT: Reid & Nygren, 1988).

The NASA-TLX workload is measured after the task, using ratings on six scales:

- mental demand
- physical demand
- temporal demand

- performance
- effort
- frustration level.

The respondent then indicates the relative importance or impact of each of the workload dimensions.

SWAT measures comprise three domains

- mental effort
- time load
- psychological stress.

Paper and pencil and computer-administered versions are available for both NASA-TLX and SWAT. For both, workload can be estimated by combining the ratings on the scales with the relative impact (weighting) score. Moroney, Biers and Eggemeier (1995) have argued that the unweighted ratings are as accurate as the more time-consuming weighted methodology. Ratings should occur within about 15 minutes of task/work completion.

Tattersall (2000) suggested that an alternative method is to use workload ratings during work (at given intervals) rather than after a work period. TLX and SWAT can both be used in this way, as can the Instantaneous Self-Assessment (ISA) measure developed by Tattersall and Foord (1996). It gives a global estimate of workload on a five-point scale using a verbal or manual response.

Physiological measures

Although not of immediate practical importance, physiological measures are based on the assumption that as workload increases and greater effort is invested, there will be an increase in psycho-physiological responses (i.e. an increase in central nervous system activity).

It is argued that such measures are more objective and less invasive, and can be used continuously (e.g. heart rate monitoring) without interfering with the primary task (Veltman & Gaillard, 1996). Physiological measures are also sensitive to physical activity and emotional states (Tattersall, 2000). Techniques include measures of brain activity, pupil dilation, cardiac activity and eye blinks.

Sleep loss

Sleep loss: how does it affect performance?

Problems with sleep are probably the commonest and most serious complaints of shift workers. Sleep loss can be an outcome of stressful work conditions (including night and shift work) and it can also be a source of fatigue and stress. Sleep loss in relation to work scheduling has been implicated as one of the links between stress and clinical care (Firth-Cozens, 1993). Night (and morning) shift work is typically associated with shorter sleep duration with premature awakening, feelings of getting too little sleep and not being rested after sleep. Obtaining less and, sometimes, little or no sleep in a 24-hour period results in acute partial sleep deprivation which affects performance and safety (Akerstedt, 1990). Acute partial sleep deficit can generally be countered by adequate periods of sleep.

Research studies report that doctors perceive that their medical performance suffers as a result of sleep loss during night work and persists during the day following the night duty (Arnetz et al., 1986). Sleep loss can result in more negative mood states and the fatigued individual may be disinclined to apply effort to tasks, resulting in reduced performance (Engel et al., 1987; Dinges & Kribbs, 1991). Mental fatigue may lead to inability to produce the right quantity and quality of work (Craig & Cooper, 1992).

The desire for sleep can conflict with responsibilities for patient care. Doctors use naps as a way of compensating for sleep loss. They may not use caffeine if their work-rest pattern is ill-defined, as caffeine may interfere with the ability to sleep when the opportunity arises.

Problems with sleep are probably the commonest complaints of shift workers. Night (and morning) shift work is typically associated with shorter sleep duration. A review of scientific and technical reports on the 24-hour distribution of medical incidents and performance failures revealed that more serious incidents were caused or made worse by human error at times when sleepiness was high and alertness and performance capability were depleted (Mitler et al., 1988).

A bimodal potential for reduced safety over the 24-hour period roughly parallels physiologically based sleep rhythms (Lavie, 1991). Safety is more likely to be compromised between approximately 0100h to 0600h and, to a lesser extent, 1400h to 1800h (the 'post-lunch dip').

Folkard (1997) reiterated these points but also suggested non-circadian time on shift effects on performance.

Not only is the sleep of shift workers disturbed but so too is wakefulness. For example, sleepiness at night often reaches levels at which wakefulness simply cannot be maintained (Torsvall et al., 1989). There may be increased lapses of attention, increased error and microsleeps of which the night worker may be completely unaware (Dinges & Kribbs, 1991; Johnson, 1982). Repeated experience of acute sleep deprivation does not appear to inoculate against its effects (Webb and Levy, 1984). The only real solution to loss of sleep is achieving adequate amounts of it.

Sleep loss may contribute to greater fatigue when the following occur:

- the length of a task increases
- difficulty of mental and physical demands increases
- memory required to undertake a task increases
- a task was recently learned
- the task is externally paced (Johnson and Naitoh, 1974).

The propensity to fall asleep at work at night can be exaggerated if the shift worker is suffering from partial sleep deprivation (Lavie, 1991). At greater levels of sleepiness under acute sleep loss the brain becomes more dependent on the environment to maintain alertness. Consequently, exposure to performance tasks requiring sustained attention may accelerate the sleep-deprived brain's tendency to move towards sleep (Dinges, 1989b; 1991).

Work with flight simulators has shown that flying performance at night may be reduced to a level corresponding to having a 0.05% blood alcohol level such as that following moderate alcohol consumption (Klein *et al.*, 1970). Lapses may result in the employee not performing their job appropriately and failing to avoid hazards. People may be unaware of these lapses and associated performance decrements.

Despite some conflicting evidence (Firth-Cozens, 1992; Jex *et al.*, 1991) there is support for the view that mood, psychological wellbeing, performance and safety are impaired by working long hours and/or suffering sleep loss (e.g. Firth-Cozens, 1987; Hurwitz *et al.*, 1987; McManus Lockwood & Cruikshank, 1977; Dinges and Kribbs, 1991; Bonnett & Arand, 1994).*

The research on sleep loss effects on clinical work indicates a number of effects. For instance:

- Sleepiness measured at three-hourly intervals through night duties was at its peak between 0300 and 0600. Doctors used naps as a way of compensating for sleep lost as a result of night duties (Arnetz *et al.*, 1990).
- Deterioration in British doctors' job efficiency has been related to sleep loss (Wilkinson, Tyler & Varey, 1975).
- Sleep-deprived doctors were reported to have experienced a significant increase in the numbers of errors made in reading ECG output (Friedman, Bigger & Kornfeld, 1971).
- Performing optimally immediately on waking from sleep is problematic. Sleep inertia (a form of 'warm-up decrement') experienced immediately after a period of sleep can affect performance because it can take some time (up to 30 minutes) to dissipate (Dinges, 1989a; Stampi, 1989).
- Night work-related sleep deprivation (4 hours or less sleep per night) resulted in increased fatigue and decreased motivation but had no effect on learning of short and longer tasks (Browne *et al.*, 1994).
- A significant decline in cognitive task performance (training examination performance) was associated with greater sleep loss on the night before the test (Jacques, Lynch & Samkoff, 1990).
- An acute decrement in sleep duration of 2–4 hours in medical settings could be reflected by performance decrements. The fatigued individual may be disinclined to apply any more effort to a task, resulting in performance decrements (Bonnet, 1994; Hartley, 1974; Wilkinson, 1968).
- Mental fatigue may involve not only an apparent inability to produce the right quantity of work, but also an inability to do the right kind of work (Craig & Cooper, 1992).
- A study of Swedish surgeons reported that 8% of doctors felt that their medical performance suffered during on-call night work while another 11% stated that their performance was moderately affected. During the day following the night duty the figures were 17% and 19% respectively (Arnetz *et al.*, 1986).

---

* Inconsistency in the findings on work hours and sleep loss effects could be related to the different ways individual people respond to work. This view is supported by the shift work research literature. Harma (1993) reported that people differ considerably in their capacities to tolerate shift and night work as a function of situational, biological and psychological characteristics. Tanz & Charrow (1993) reported that 'functional' differences resulted in less effective work practices, inefficiency and the creation of extra work, e.g. it is possible that some doctors sleep less than they could (with detrimental effects). Increasing/improving sleep could alter perceptions of workload, improve satisfaction and contribute to better performance.

- Doctors are aware of the potential risk of deterioration in performance capability and decision making (Arnetz *et al.*, 1986; Smith *et al.*, 1999).

In a review of studies from 1970 to 1990, Samkoff and Jacques (1991) concluded that sleep deprivation and fatigue are related to decreased mood and poorer attitudes. Acute sleep loss was also related to decreased vigilance but not to dexterity, reaction time or short-term memory tasks. This suggests that doctors compensate for sleep loss in crisis or novel situations. However, sleep-deprived doctors may be more prone to errors on routine, repetitive tasks and those tasks needing sustained attention (which form a substantial proportion of PRHOs' workload).

A review of the effects of on-call schedules on doctors' sleep, performance and mood (Bonnett & Arand, 1994) found that impaired performance related to sleep loss was more likely for reasoning tasks, for non-stimulating tasks and less-experienced doctors.

That on-call duties interfere with sleep is of major concern because the amount of sleep available when on call is highly variable and the desire for sleep can conflict with responsibilities for patient care.

What are the existing methods for the assessment of sleep loss and its impact on the performance of a doctor?

Sleep is probably the area of a shift worker's life associated with the greatest disruption. As well as primary measures or estimates of sleep actually achieved, a number of other secondary sleep- and sleepiness-related measures are described.

- The *Stanford Sleepiness Scale* (Hoddes *et al.*, 1973) is a 7-point Likert-type scale with anchor points ranging from 'very alert' to 'very sleepy'. Respondents choose the descriptors that best describe their feeling of sleepiness at a particular moment. It can be used as a concurrent state measure at regular intervals and/or a retrospective measure.
- The *Epworth Sleepiness Scale* (Johns, 1991): A self-report tool that contains a description of eight different real life situations. Respondents rate their likelihood of falling asleep in each of the listed situations. Typically used as a general sleepiness measure.
- *Visual Analogue Scales* (VAS) may be used to index sleepiness. Typically, it would consist of a 100 mm line with anchor points of, say, 'very alert' at one end and 'very sleepy' at the other. Respondents mark the line at a point they believe to be a reflection of their current state of alertness.

Other physiological tests including actigraphy (measuring levels of ambulatory bodily activity, from sleep sedentary to highly active) and assessment methods used in sleep laboratories are available but are of less practical usefulness.

Shiftwork and its effects

Shift scheduling is now a pervasive feature of the occupational landscape that has many implications for performance, health and safety. 'Shift work' refers to the extension of work time beyond 'normal' office hours, requiring two or more teams, firms or 'shifts' to provide operational cover. It has also come to represent irregular work hours, and, for some, permanent evening or night duty (Akerstedt, 1990; Smith *et al.*, 1998a).

It is common to find that many staff work regularly beyond the official hours for which they are contracted. Consequently, difficulties associated with work hours (as these contribute to 'workload' exposure) may be increased in doctors regardless of their work schedule. The out-of-hours (outside the normal 0800–1700) work period and long-hours workload traditionally covered by doctors on call has been highlighted (Ferguson, Shandall & Griffith, 1994; Leslie *et al.*, 1990).

Non-standard work hours, especially when regular night duty is involved, can harbour the potential for serious consequences. There can be both direct and indirect effects. Direct effects include disruption to the body clock, sleep, alertness, mood and performance. Indirect effects include disruption to family and social life, which may exacerbate already stressful circumstances (Scott, 1990; Smith *et al.*, 1998b). The pressures of high workload, downturns in psychological state and increase in 'risky' coping behaviours may be amplified if a doctor finds herself/ himself working an uncompromising work schedule.

Research suggests that the devil is in the detail. Relatively shorter work hours are not necessarily a good or a bad thing; the crucial issue is how the hours/shifts are configured in relation to operational constraints, demands, and social require-ments. Changes to the configuration of on-call and shift rotas, combined with improvements to support staff provision and training in intervention strategies, can help doctors to cope more effectively with shift work. The configuration issue is important because, even in apparently better shift systems, doctors may still be required to work very long hours in some weeks.

Perhaps the over-riding issue is that of potential high fatigue levels exacerbated by sleep loss and high work demands. A study of physicians working night call duty showed effects on sleepiness with residual effects (elevated sleepiness) persisting after the on-call duty period (Arnetz, Akerstedt & Anderzen, 1990).

Professionalism and the high stakes associated with failure mean that compensa-tory effort is invested in an attempt to maintain satisfactory clinical performance. This can serve to counter the debilitating effects of sleep loss and fatigue. However, there comes a point when tiredness is so great that any task performance or treatment decision can be degraded. People differ in their capacity to tolerate shift and night work rotas. Part of the difference relates to the level and sophistication of personal strategies that can be deployed. In light of this, it is also feasible to provide training in appropriate interventions to help medical staff cope more readily with their work schedules (in conjunction with the judicious configuration of working hours).

The National Health Service will be required to reduce the number of hours worked. Whilst this would reduce the potential for adverse effects on staff working long hours, the risk of problems associated with shiftworking could still remain.

How does shift work affect performance?

The potential adverse effects of shift working are well chronicled (Colquhoun *et al.*, 1996; Folkard and Monk, 1985; Scott, 1990; Waterhouse, Folkard and Minors, 1992). Outcomes fall into a number of areas:

- biological disruption to physiological processes, including the sleep-wake cycle (Tepas & Mahan, 1989)

- impairment of physical health and psychological wellbeing (Akerstedt, 1990; Waterhouse, Folkard & Minors, 1992)
- reduced alertness, performance and safety (Akerstedt, 1991; Folkard, 1997; Nurminen, 1998)
- consequences in terms of productivity, moonlighting, sickness absence and turnover (Smith *et al.*, 1998), depending on work schedule configuration
- interference with social and domestic life (Barton, Aldridge & Smith, 1998; Fischer *et al.*, 1993; Volger *et al.*, 1988).

Shift workers may engage in more 'risky' coping behaviours that contribute to impairment to health, e.g. increased smoking, caffeine, alcohol, or drug use and changed eating habits (Kivimaki *et al.*, 2001; Knutsson, 1989; Haider *et al.*, 1981; Olsson, Kandolin & Kauppinintoropainen, 1990).

The extent to which shift work affects the individual depends largely upon the job being done, characteristics of the individual (personal coping resources, personality), organisational and social environments and features of the shift system (Harma, 1993; Knauth, 1996).

What are the existing methods for the assessment of the impact of shift work on the performance of a doctor?

The primary methodology for studying shift work effects has been the use of self-report instruments.

Shift work-related self-report questionnaire components

Information on the following factors is typically gathered in shift work surveys:

- biographical details
- working time details
- sleep – duration, quality
- alertness
- fatigue
- psychological wellbeing
- physical health
- social/family interference
- coping strategies
- individual differences.

Motivation and compensatory effort

Even extremely tired individuals can demonstrate high levels of performance on complex tasks that stimulate interest (Hockey, 1996; Craig & Cooper, 1992). There can be a tendency to underestimate the ability of individuals to motivate themselves to overcome the effects of sleep loss or fatigue on performance. For example, the capacity of doctors to 'rally in certain circumstances' has been noted.

Dinges and Kribbs (1991) noted that sleep loss may affect the 'willingness to perform' rather than the capacity to perform. By using a variety of motivational variables such as incentives, signals, reminders, feedback and exhortations, performance levels can be raised in sleep-deprived individuals. However, this motivated effort cannot be sustained for long if workload is maintained at a high level and:

- task demands persist or
- new tasks compete for significant attention or
- the task is contained within other continuous work.

Motivation may be used to sustain performance at near-baseline levels if the amount of sleep achieved has not been reduced below 50% of typical sleep duration and if the period of wakefulness following sleep deprivation does not exceed 24 hours (Dinges *et al.*, 1987).

In a study of cognitive performance, night work and workload in doctors, Deary and Tait (1987) reported that some tired doctors performed better than their more alert colleagues. They also noted that tasks that were more closely related to actual job performance were not detrimentally affected by the more adverse conditions.

Outcomes of surgery have been examined in relation to surgeons' levels of sleep deprivation. Doctors who operated during the day after a 24-hour on-call period were considered sleep-deprived. However, no significant change in post-operative complication incidence was found in relation to level of surgeon sleep deprivation (Haynes *et al.*, 1995).

No significant performance decrements were observed in junior doctors, even when sleep loss increased up to 72 hours (Ford & Wentz, 1986).

Intervention to increase or improve personal coping strategies is possible and may be a consideration for doctors in training. Jones *et al.* (1988) reported the success of a hospital-wide stress-management programme in reducing medication errors. The benefits of such intervention have been indicated by a reduction in malpractice claims in hospitals that had implemented stress-management training (Firth-Cozens, 1998).

The effects of shift work: what interventions are possible and how effective are they?

A range of coping strategies, training and information can be offered to shift workers to improve their performance. The challenge to employing organisations is to identify and implement effective, multifaceted strategies to equip shift workers to combat the demands of their rotas.

Individual differences in tolerance of shift working mean that it is not possible to offer a panacea for all shift work 'ills'. There is no 'ideal' shift system but only less bad ones, which cater for the particular circumstances prevailing in an organisation.

Nevertheless, a range of interventions is possible including:

- changing the rota
- providing information, training and counselling on coping strategies, including:
  - sleep strategies
  - napping
  - meal timing and content

- – exercise and conditioning
- – counselling
- drugs and hormones
- screening and shift worker selection
- changing the work environment.

Changing the rota

Changing work rotas is the common organisational 'catch-all' approach to minimising sleep loss, fatigue, stress and workload-related outcomes. This was a large part of the motivation behind the New Deal on working hours for junior doctors introduced in 1991. It aimed to reduce hours of work and to improve overall working conditions while maintaining clinical and educational standards. There have only been a small number of commentaries and studies (Barrett, 1995; Fisher *et al.*, 1994). The outcome of this initiative, at least in terms of work hours, has tended to be equivocal at best.

No detrimental effects on patient care or educational standards were reported after the introduction of a partial shift rota that reduced weekly hours to an average of 64 hours/week. The areas of improvement were reported to be: reduced hours, shorter periods of continuous duty, better quality off-duty hours, no chronic fatigue, improved family and social life, and shorter weekend duties (Vassallo *et al.*, 1992). However, there were reservations. These included the timing and nature of the 'cover' shift and problems with night duties such as disruption to social life, impairment of firms' 'team spirit' and interference with continuity of care. The partial shift system was deemed applicable but the house surgeons that participated in the study were equally divided in their preferences between the on-call and partial shift systems.

A partial shift system introduced for a group of pre-registration house surgeons was noted to be generally applicable, but the doctors' wellbeing and performance effectiveness were not systematically studied (Hartley & Rothera, 1994).

In another study, shift rotas had a negative effect on job satisfaction, psychological wellbeing and, importantly, on training (Kapur & House, 1998).

Kelty, Duffy and Cooper (1999) explored the effects of a reduction in on-call duty over a 6-year period (1990–1995) on trainees' experience of relatively uncommon emergencies in cardiothoracic surgery. They suggested that the New Deal arrangement would reduce trainees' experience in higher specialist training by 50% and that there should be a mechanism to allow trainees to be on call more often in order to obtain adequate specialist training.

Research by Hale *et al.* (1995) studied two groups of house surgeons that worked 6 weeks on partial shifts and 6 weeks on a 'one in six' on-call rota in a balanced design. Doctors expected that both partial shifts and on-call duty would result in equal levels of anxiety at work but that the partial shifts would reduce fatigue levels. Anxiety levels were greater on the partial shift system. A particular concern was that house officers 'felt isolated' from colleagues during night shifts. Fatigue levels were similar on both schedules. A majority of house officers reported impairment to communication with patients and senior colleagues when on the partial shift system. Educational value was considered but the results were equivocal.

Providing information, training and counselling on coping strategies

Educational programmes for shift workers are often advocated but rarely implemented. Shift workers tend to develop their own ways of coping, either intentionally or by accident. Interestingly, in addition to coping guidance, many shift workers want 'the rest of the world' (i.e. managers, day workers, general public and families) to be made aware of the potential effects of shift working.

The challenge is to bring less experienced shift workers 'up to speed' sooner by providing guidance about effective interventions that they might try or adapt. Employers can help by producing coping guidance documentation for trainee health professionals.

Educators can help by raising awareness of the risks to clinical performance, personal health and safety of shift work and by providing proactive advice on coping with shift working, workload, sleep loss and fatigue.

Sleep strategies

Achieving adequate sleep is a major problem for shift workers but there are no magic ways to fall asleep quickly or to sleep well. A range of non drug-based interventions is possible (Morin *et al.*, 1994), including:

- **Stimulus control:** Comprising a set of instructions for procedures that are designed to reduce behaviours incompatible with gaining good sleep.
- **Sleep restriction:** This involves limiting the time spent in bed to the actual amount of sleep achieved.
- **Relaxation strategies:** These interventions are designed to reduce bodily or mental activation. A range of strategies is readily available in book and audiotape format. Training in relaxation methods is possible. Mental relaxation techniques appear to be as effective as physically based methods.

Research has found stimulus control and sleep restriction to be the most effective single-use interventions.

Sleep hygiene education may be an effective preventive strategy and is concerned with providing information about the effects of:

- circadian rhythms
- sleep deprivation
- sleep scheduling
- sleep habits
- diet
- exercise
- naps
- stimulants
- smoking
- alcohol
- ambient temperature
- environmental noise.

Napping

Napping any time tends to be beneficial, for even 15 minutes structured into a lunch break can affect subsequent alertness and performance (Takahashi *et al.*, 2003) and napping during night shifts can help post-shift recovery (Matsumoto & Harada, 1994). The timing of a nap determines whether it is aimed at preventing anticipated decreases in alertness and increases in fatigue (pre-emptive naps), or at making up for the lowered alertness and heightened fatigue already experienced (replacement or maintenance naps). Naps prior to a period of sleep loss have been found to benefit both performance and alertness, and reduce fatigue during the night. Naps taken during the work shift can compensate for partial sleep deprivation, but there should always be a post-nap waking-up period 'built-in' (Bonnet & Arand, 1994).

Meal timing and content

Digestive problems are common complaints in shift workers. Night workers typically sleep through at least one 'normal' daytime meal and eat at night when day workers sleep. Shift workers may also change what they eat at night (e.g. to high sugar content snacking, and sometimes high fat meals). Intervention has been suggested in terms of:

- the programmed use of meals and social activity as time-cues
- different types of meals to promote conditions for encouraging/inhibiting the biochemicals associated with wakefulness and sleep (Ehret, 1980; Romon-Rousseaux *et al.*, 1987)
- the structured use of caffeinated drinks and similar agents.

Exercise and conditioning

There is evidence to suggest that improving the physical condition of shift workers can either increase their tolerance or increase their rate of adjustment. Physical training may not only improve fitness but has been associated with lowered fatigue on night shift, decreased general musculo-skeletal discomfort and increased sleep durations after evening shifts (Harma *et al.*, 1988a; Harma *et al.*, 1988b). Maximal oxygen consumption and muscle strength were considered to be the most important influences on the observed improvements (Harma *et al.*, 1988b,c).

Counselling

Counselling sessions designed to improve the sleep behaviour of shift workers have resulted in an increase in the sleep durations of participants (Carlson, 1991). It is a promising focused intervention that has proven to be effective, at least in the medium term (Taylor, 1994). It appears to be capable of reducing disruption to circadian and social rhythms. 'In-house' shift work experts could be trained to give practical advice to shift workers. Occupational health practitioners could provide information to shift workers during medical check-ups.

Drugs and hormones

Typical medical treatment for sleep disturbance is the prescription of drugs such as benzodiazepines (Rosa *et al.*, 1990). In the short term they reduce sleep latency, reduce the number and duration of awakenings, increase total sleep time and improve sleep efficiency. However, long-term use (even for two or three weeks) can lead to problems of alteration of sleep stages, residual effects during daytime, development of tolerance, dependence, and 'rebound' insomnia (Morin, Culbert & Schwartz, 1994).

Human rhythms can also be influenced by the regulated ingestion of the hormone melatonin, a natural sleep-related substance produced by the pineal gland during the hours of darkness (Folkard, Arendt & Clark, 1993). Melatonin (which is unavailable in the UK) has sedative properties and may help achieve better sleep following night duty but its long-term effects are unclear.

Night workers and rotating shift workers have reported greater use of stimulants such as caffeine (in tablet form as well as in beverages). Programmed caffeine intake in conjunction with the use of other strategies may prove effective in helping adaptation to night work. The stimulant Modafinil has been proposed for potential use in shift/night working conditions as an aid to alertness. Caldwell *et al.* (2000) have reported that the drug attenuates sleep loss effects on performance and improves subjective states. With the need for only small doses, there are advantages over amphetamines because of reported minimal side effects (Lyons & French, 1991).

Alcohol ingestion is commonly used as a sleep aid by shift workers. However, although it helps induce sleep, it has been shown to disturb certain stages of sleep and can cause sleep fragmentation, not least because the shift worker has to rise to go to the toilet.

Screening and shift worker selection

Individual tolerance of shift work varies considerably (Harma, 1993; Scott & Ladou, 1990). Although individual doctors, for example established general practitioners, may be able to 'opt out' of out-of-hours shift work, many do not have the choice. Because of staffing requirements and other constraints, medical employers rarely consider aptitude for shift work when selecting employees.

Factors that could be considered when selecting individuals for shift work include:

- **Age:** Shift workers tend to become less tolerant of their schedules as they get older.
- **Gender:** Women tend to sacrifice their own sleep and wellbeing to attend to the needs of their families or partners.
- **Sleep habits:** Flexible sleepers appear to tolerate night work more effectively.
- **'Morningness':** A behavioural/psychological factor theoretically tied to the peak of circadian rhythms. Some people have extreme peaks of activity in the morning ('larks') or the evening ('owls'). Morningness is an expression of early peaking of the circadian rhythms, including physical signs such as body temperature. Typically, morning people prefer to get up relatively earlier, work, be active earlier in the day, and to go to bed/sleep relatively early. This nature is in conflict with staying awake and active on shifts that run through the night.

Human beings tend to become more morning-oriented as they age, contributing to older individuals' poorer tolerance of shift and night work.

- **Amplitude of circadian rhythms:** Appears to be related to shift work tolerance. Smaller rhythm amplitudes (which can also occur as we get older) appear to be linked to poorer long-term tolerance to shift work.
- **Psychological characteristics:** Beliefs, attitudes and motivation will have an influence on coping with a rota, as will the resourcefulness of the person (the personal coping 'tool-kit' built-up by the worker through life experiences).

Screening should take place prior to commencing shift work (this could be wholly, or partly, in the form of a questionnaire in addition to a physical examination). In addition to the factors listed above, screening could cover areas such as medical disorders, symptoms of sleep deprivation, family or other social conflicts, weight loss, general nutritional status and the use of caffeinated drinks, alcohol, sleeping pills and cigarettes. The results could help highlight those individuals who might have difficulty with shift work, or be unsuitable. A number of contraindications for shift work can be identified (Scott & Ladou, 1990). These fall into two categories:

- Those that may be aggravated by shift work, e.g. extreme 'morningness', insomnia, age 45+.
- Medical conditions that a physician may feel warrant a recommendation to restrict someone from undertaking shift work, e.g. epilepsy requiring medication, coronary artery disease, chronic depression, pregnancy.

Monitoring should be maintained at regular intervals appropriate to the individual (based on the risks identified through the pre-shift work screening). Ill effects caused or exacerbated by shift work may take several years to manifest themselves. Many shift workers habituate to their rota and accept that they may feel worse at certain times as part of the job, but they could ignore or miss problems that could require medical or other attention. Commitment to long-term checks should be maintained.

Changing the work environment

Even when the most appropriate 24-hour shift rota is implemented, there is still the requirement for people to work at night. Bright light affects the timing of body rhythms (Czeisler, 1995). It offers a tangible and effective method to help shift workers feel better and operate more effectively at night (Czeisler *et al.*, 1990; Foret *et al.*, 1996). Bright light technology is an intervention that can be used alongside judicious choice of shift rota, and other guidance. Bright light exposure at night has been linked to better physical fitness, lower tiredness and sleepiness, a more balanced sleep pattern and higher performance efficiency (Morisseau *et al.*, 1996).

Other interventions

There is a need for a step-change in attitude to sleep loss and fatigue such that it becomes unacceptable for doctors (and other health professionals) to try to work under conditions of severe sleepiness and fatigue and high work demands. That is, there should be concerted efforts to promote cultural change – to value sleep and more tolerable work rotas – founded on research and education.

If necessary, we should consider changing trainee doctors' (and other health service professionals') patterns of work hours. The intention would be to provide intervention at an organisational level to combat sleep loss and workload effects. Any change regime should have at its heart the participation of those whose working conditions are being affected. Appendix 1 offers an example of how such a change process might be organised. These recommendations assume that the factors combine or interact, and that addressing problems in one area could have a knock-on effect upon other areas, especially where sleep is improved. They echo similar moves in the United States to address the issues of doctors' fatigue and working hours, where concerted and large-scale research is being undertaken to help improve conditions (Lamberg, 2002). The recommendations are not mutually exclusive and bear further development with regard to making specific recommendations. They are intended to provide a stepping stone to reducing the negative impact of workload, sleep loss and shift working upon clinical performance and clinicians' health.

At national and local level, doctors (and other health professionals) should be involved at every stage of the decision-making process that holds implications for their clinical practice, personal health and safety. Real participation is crucial to the success of interventions.

Questions for further research

There is a need for improved measurement criteria with which to identify the current status of workload, sleep loss and the effects of working hours (and their interaction) on a national (representative) basis, and within diverse settings in the healthcare sector. This would include identification of the work rotas currently operating.

Research could also map out the pattern of impacts of workload, sleep deprivation and shift work on doctors' training, patient care, doctors' health, professional conduct and economic considerations and help to identify causal relationships between the factors and outcomes for patients, doctors, and healthcare organisations.

Conclusion

The interest in possible deterioration in the performance of medical professionals in general and doctors in particular as a consequence of the organisation of work hours is not a new phenomenon; there has been research into the topic over the past three or four decades. Despite this research effort, it remains difficult to identify precisely how long a person should work, given the incentives prevalent in the clinical domain and the resourcefulness of human beings.

Nevertheless, there may be a point, in terms of work hours, beyond which it is unwise to ask, or require, a medical practitioner to work and expect optimal performance. It is also worrying that despite the extensive of scientific literature on the effects of shift and night working, much of it in relation to medical and nursing staff, there remains a lack of current knowledge about the impact of new and persisting work rotas upon doctors nationwide. Furthermore, there has been little concerted effort in testing, and providing the doctors, nursing staff and other healthcare workers with, a set of tangible interventions targeted at combating the negative impact of shift and night work.

Appendix 1: stages to be considered in shift rota change

The stages are not mutually exclusive and a degree of parallel activity would be envisaged.

Planning and preparation

Project team established to include shift workers, employers and scientific expertise.
Clarify powers and competence.
Ensure communication between all levels.
Define aims and terms of reference.
Check aims against legislation and collective agreements.
Identify shift worker and organisational preferences/goals.
Establish plan for organisation of changeover and time frame of programme.
Generate different shift rotas and staffing levels.
Refer to scientific knowledge base regarding ergonomic principles as well as team knowledge.
Identify measurement criteria.
Plan data collection.

Analysis

Test group and control group selected.
Further consultation and discussion with employees/unions involved.
Thorough analysis of present state – both inside and outside the organisation.
Comparison of proposed rota(s) with existing knowledge.
Survey/study of current state relative to work rotas, sleep loss and workload.
First/basic versions of possible rotas developed.

Design

Consultation with employees/unions, employers, scientific experts.
Reference to ergonomic principles (shift work research).
Improvements to models of alternative shift systems developed.
Details of rota(s) formulated.
Vote on rota to test.

Testing

Test new work rota for agreed and fixed time period.
Compare within change group and between change and no-change groups.
Monitor and discuss impact on management and workforce.
Survey employees on new rota and comparison group(s).
Consider potential for amendments where feasible.

Implementation and evaluation

Modify the system where improvements can be made.
Agree the system and its parameters, including financial (with interested agencies).

Vote on implementation.

Make decision about whether or not to proceed with full-scale introduction.

Implement.

Evaluate regularly against predetermined criteria (e.g. self-report on sleep, workload, stress, etc.; clinical effectiveness; patient care; sickness absence; turnover; economic factors).

Promote culture of continuous improvement.

References

Akerstedt T (1990) Psychological and psychophysiological effects of shift work. *Scandinavian Journal of Work, Environment and Health*. 16(Suppl 1): 67–73.

Akerstedt T (1991) Sleepiness at work: effects of irregular work hours. In: TH Monk (ed.) *Sleep, Sleepiness and Performance*. John Wiley & Sons, Chichester, pp. 129–52.

Aretz AJ, Johannsen C and Obser K (1996) An empirical validation of subjective workload ratings. In: *Proceedings of the Human Factors and Ergonomics Society 40th Annual Meeting*. Human Factors and Ergonomics Society, Santa Monica, CA, pp. 91–5.

Arnetz BB, Andreasson D, Strandberg M, Eneroth P and Kallner A (1986) Physicians work environment: Psychosocial, physical and physiological data from a structured in-depth interview and biochemical assessment of general surgeons and general practitioners. *Stress Reports* No. 187; Karolinska Institute, Stockholm. (Swedish with English summary.)

Arnetz BB, Akerstedt T and Anderzen I (1990) Sleepiness in physicians on night call duty. *Work and Stress*. 4(1): 71–3.

Arnold J, Cooper C and Robertson I (1995) *Work Psychology: understanding human behaviour in the workplace* (2e). Pitman, London.

Barrett A (1995) Junior doctors' hours: Beat the clock. *Nursing Standard*. 10(11): 18–19.

Barton J, Aldridge J and Smith P (1998) The emotional impact of shift work on the children of shift workers. *Scandinavian Journal of Work, Environment and Health*. 24(Suppl 3): 146–50.

Bonnet MH (1994) Sleep deprivation. In: MH Kryger, T Roth and WC Dement (eds) *Principles and Practice of Sleep Medicine* (2e). WB Saunders, Philadelphia, ch.5.

Bonnet MH and Arand DL (1994) The use of prophylactic naps and caffeine to maintain performance during a continuous operation. *Ergonomics*. 37(6): 1009–20.

Browne BJ *et al.* (1994) Influence of sleep deprivation on learning among surgical house staff and medical students. *Surgery*. 115(5): 604–10.

Caldwell JA *et al.* (2000) A double-blind placebo-controlled investigation of the efficacy of Modafinil for sustaining the alertness and performance of aviators: a helicopter simulator study. *Psychopharmacology*. 150(3): 272–82.

Carlson ML (1991) Sleep management training: An intervention programme to improve the sleep of shift workers. *Sleep Research*. 20: 115.

Casali JG and Wierwille WW (1983) A comparison of rating scale, secondary-task, physiological and primary-task workload estimation techniques in a simulated flight task emphasizing communications load. *Human Factors*. 25(6): 623–41.

Colquhoun WP *et al.* (1996) *Shift Work Problems and Solutions*. Peter Lang, Frankfurt am Main, Berlin.

Craig A and Cooper RE (1992) Symptoms of acute and chronic fatigue. In: AP Smith and DM Jones (eds) *Handbook of Human Performance*. Academic Press, London, pp. 289–339.

Czeisler CA (1995) The effect of light on the human circadian pacemaker. In: DJ Chadwick and K Ackrill (eds) *Circadian Clocks and Their Adjustment*. Ciba Foundation Symposium 183. John Wiley & Sons, Chichester, pp. 254–302.

Czeisler CA *et al.* (1990) Exposure to bright light and darkness to treat physiologic maladaptation to night work. *New England Journal of Medicine.* **322**(18): 1253–9.

Damos DL (1991) *Multiple-task Performance.* Taylor and Francis, London.

Deary IJ and Tait R (1987) Effects of sleep disruption on cognitive performance and mood in medical house officers. *BMJ.* **295**(6612): 1513–16.

Dinges DF (1989a) Napping patterns and effects in human adults. In: DF Dinges and RJ Broughton (eds) *Sleep and Alertness: chronobiological, behavioral and medical aspects of napping.* Raven Press, New York, pp. 171–204.

Dinges DF (1989b) The nature of sleepiness: causes, contexts and consequences. In: AJ Stunkard and A Baum (eds) *Eating, Sleeping and Sex.* Perspectives in Behavioral Medicine Series. Lawrence Erlbaum Associates, Hillsdale, NJ, pp. 147–79.

Dinges DF (1991) Probing the limits of functional capability: The effects of sleep loss on short-duration tasks. In: RJ Broughton and RD Ogilvie (eds) *Sleep, Arousal and Performance: a tribute to Bob Wilkinson.* Proceedings of a Conference held in May 1990. Birkhauser, Boston, pp. 176–88.

Dinges DF and Kribbs NB (1991) Performing while sleepy: effects of experimentally-induced sleepiness. In: TH Monk (ed.) *Sleep, Sleepiness and Performance.* John Wiley & Sons, Chichester, pp. 97–128.

Dinges DF *et al.* (1987) Temporal placement of a nap for alertness: contributions of circadian phase and prior wakefulness. *Sleep.* **10**(4): 313–29.

Ehret CF (1980) New approaches to chronohygiene for the shift worker in the nuclear power industry. In: A Reinberg, N Vieux and P Andlauer (eds) *Night and Shift Work: biological and social aspects.* Proceedings of the Fifth International Symposium on night and shift work, Rouen, 12–16 May 1980. Advances in the Biosciences Series, 30. Pergamon, London, vol. 30, pp. 263–78.

Engel W, Seime R, Powell V and D'Alessandri R (1987) Clinical performance of interns after being on call. *Southern Medical Journal.* **80**: 761–3.

Ferguson C, Shandall A and Griffith G (1994) Out of hours workload of junior and senior house surgeons in a district general hospital. *Annals of the Royal College of Surgeons of England.* **76**(2 suppl): 53–6.

Firth-Cozens J (1987) Emotional distress in junior house officers. *BMJ.* **295**(6597): 533–6.

Firth-Cozens J (1992) The role of early experiences in the perception of organisational stress: fusing clinical and organisational perspectives. *Journal of Organizational and Occupational Psychology.* **65**: 61–75.

Firth-Cozens J (1993) Stress, psychological problems and clinical performance. In: C Vincent, M Ennis and RJ Audley (eds) *Medical Accidents.* Oxford University Press, Oxford, pp. 131–49.

Firth-Cozens J (1995) Sources of stress in junior doctors and general practitioners. *Yorkshire Medicine.* **7**(3): 10–13.

Firth-Cozens J (1998) Individual and organizational predictors of depression in general practitioners. *British Journal of General Practice.* **48**(435): 1647–51.

Firth-Cozens J and Greenhalgh J (1997) Doctors' perceptions of the links between stress and lowered clinical care. *Social Science and Medicine.* **44**(7): 1017–22.

Firth-Cozens J and Morrison L (1989) Sources of stress and ways of coping in junior house officers. *Stress Medicine.* **5**: 121–6.

Fischer FM *et al.* (1993) Day and shift workers' leisure time. *Ergonomics.* **36**(1–3): 43–9.

Fisher EW *et al.* (1994) Reduction in junior doctors' hours in an otolaryngology unit: effects on the 'out of hours' working patterns of all grades. *Annals of the Royal College of Surgeons of England.* **76**(5 suppl): 232–5.

Folkard S (1997) Black times: Temporal determinants of transport safety. *Accident Analysis and Prevention.* **29**(4): 417–30.

Folkard S, Arendt J and Clark M (1993) Can melatonin improve shift workers' tolerance to the night shift? Some preliminary findings. *Chronobiology International.* **10**(5): 315–20.

Folkard S and Monk TH (1985) *Hours of Work: temporal issues in work scheduling.* John Wiley & Sons, Chichester.

Ford CV (1983) Emotional distress in internship and residency: a questionnaire study. *Psychiatric Medicine.* **1**(2): 143–50.

Ford CV and Wentz DK (1986) Internship: what is stressful? *Southern Medical Journal.* **79**(5): 595–9.

Foret J *et al.* (1996) The effect on body temperature and melatonin of a 39 hour constant routine with two different light levels at night-time. *Chronobiology International.* **13**(1): 35–45.

Friedman RC, Bigger JT and Kornfeld DS (1971) The intern and sleep loss. *New England Journal of Medicine.* **285**(4): 201–3.

Geurts S, Rutte C and Peeters M (1999) Antecedents & consequences of home–work interference among medical residents. *Social Science and Medicine.* **48**(9): 1135–48.

Hale PC *et al.* (1995) Crossover trial of partial shift working and a one in six rota system for house surgeons in two teaching hospitals. *Journal of the Royal College of Surgeons of Edinburgh.* **40**(1): 55–8.

Harma M (1993) Individual differences in tolerance to shift work – a review. *Ergonomics.* **36**(1–3): 101–9.

Harma MI, Ilmarinen J and Knauth P (1988a) Physical fitness and other individual factors relating to the shift work tolerance of women. *Chronobiology International.* **54**: 417–24.

Harma MI *et al.* (1988b) Physical training intervention in female shift workers (I). The effects of intervention on fitness, fatigue, sleep and psychosomatic symptoms. *Ergonomics.* **31**(1): 39–50.

Harma MI *et al.* (1988c) Physical training intervention in female shift workers (II). The effects of intervention on the circadian rhythms of alertness, short-term memory and body temperature. *Ergonomics.* **31**(1): 51–63.

Hart SG and Staveland LE (1988) Development of a NASA TLX (Task Load Index): Results of empirical and theoretical research. In: P Hancock and N Meshkati (eds) *Human Mental Workload.* Advances in Psychology Series, 52. Elsevier, Amsterdam, pp. 139–83.

Hartley LR (1974) A comparison of continuous and distributed reduced sleep schedules. *Quarterly Journal of Experimental Psychology.* **26**(Feb): 8–14.

Hartley C and Rothera MP (1994) A new deal for ENT surgeons – the Manchester experience 1992–3. *Annals of the Royal College of Surgeons of England.* **76**(5 Suppl): 228–31.

Haynes DF *et al.* (1995) Are postoperative complications related to resident sleep deprivation? *Southern Medical Journal.* **88**(3): 283–9.

Heyworth J *et al.* (1993) Predictors of work satisfaction among SHOs during accident and emergency medical training. *Archives of Emergency Medicine.* **10**(4): 279–88.

Hockey GRJ (1996) Skill and workload. In: PB Warr (ed.) *Psychology at Work* (4e). Penguin, Harmondsworth.

Hoddes E *et al.* (1973) Quantification of sleepiness: a new approach. *Psychophysiology.* **10**(4): 431–6.

Hurwitz TA *et al.* (1987) Impaired interns and residents. *Canadian Journal of Psychiatry.* **32**(3): 165–9.

Jacques CH, Lynch JC and Samkoff JS (1990) The effects of sleep loss on cognitive performance of resident physicians. *Journal of Family Practice.* **30**(2): 223–9.

Jex SM *et al.* (1991) Behavioural consequences of job-related stress among resident physicians: the mediating role of psychological strain. *Psychological Reports.* **69**(1): 339–49.

Johns MW (1991) A new method for measuring daytime sleepiness: the Epworth Sleepiness Scale. *Sleep.* **14**(6): 540–5.

Johnson LC (1982) Sleep deprivation and performance. In: WB Webb (ed.) *Biological Rhythms, Sleep and Performance.* John Wiley & Sons, Chichester, pp. 111–41.

Jones JW *et al.* (1988) Stress and medical malpractice: organisational risk assessment and intervention. *Journal of Applied Psychology.* **73**(4): 727–35.

Kapur N and House A (1998) Improving 'new deal' shifts for junior house officers. *Hospital Medicine.* **59**(12): 960–2, 964, 966.

Kelty C, Duffy J and Cooper G (1999) Out-of-hours work in cardiothoracic surgery: implications of the New Deal and Calman for training. *Postgraduate Medical Journal.* **75**(884): 351–2.

Kivimaki M *et al.* (2001) Does shiftwork lead to poorer health habits? A comparison between women who had always done shiftwork with those who had never done shiftwork. *Work and Stress.* **15**(1): 3–13.

Klein KE *et al.* (1970) Circadian rhythm of pilots' efficiency and effects of multiple time zone travel. *Aerospace Medicine.* **41**(2): 125–32.

Knauth P (1996) Designing better shift systems. *Applied Ergonomics.* **27**(1): 39–44.

Lamberg L (2002) Long hours, little sleep: bad medicine for physicians in training? *JAMA.* **287**(3): 303–6.

Lavie P (1991) The 24-hour sleep propensity function (SPF): practical and theoretical implications. In: TH Monk (ed.) *Sleep, Sleepiness and Performance.* John Wiley & Sons, Chichester, pp. 65–93.

Leslie PJ *et al.* (1990) Hours, volume and type of work of pre-registration house officers. *BMJ.* **300**(6731): 1038–41.

Lewittes LR and Marshall VW (1989) Fatigue and concerns about quality of care among Ontario interns and residents. *Canadian Medical Association Journal.* **140**(1): 21–4.

Lyons TJ and French J (1991) Modafinil the unique properties of a new stimulant. *Aviation, Space, and Environmental Medicine.* **62**(5): 432–5.

Matsumoto K and Harada M (1994) The effect of night-time naps on recovery from fatigue following night work. *Ergonomics.* **37**(5): 899–907.

McCue JD (1985) The distress of internship: causes and prevention. *New England Journal of Medicine.* **312**(7): 449–52.

McManus IC, Lockwood DN and Cruikshank JK (1977) The preregistration year: chaos by consensus. *The Lancet.* **1**(8008): 413–17.

Mitler MM *et al.* (1988) Catastrophes, sleep and public policy. *Sleep.* **11**(1): 100–9.

Morales IJ, Peters SG and Afessa B (2003) Hospital mortality rate and length of stay in patients admitted at night to the intensive care unit. *Critical Care Medicine.* **31**(3): 858–63.

Morin CM, Culbert JP and Schwartz SM (1994) Nonpharmacological interventions for insomnia: a meta-analysis of treatment efficacy. *American Journal of Psychiatry.* **151**(8): 1172–80.

Morisseau D, Persensky JJ, Sebrosky J and Mackinnon J (1996) Proposed article for *Nuclear News.* Unpublished manuscript/personal communication.

Moroney WF, Biers DW and Eggemeier FT (1995) Some measurement and methodological considerations in the application of subjective workload measurement techniques. *International Journal of Aviation Psychology.* **5**(1): 87–106.

Murray RM (1977) Psychiatric illness in male doctors and controls: an analysis of Scottish hospitals in-patient data. *British Journal of Psychiatry.* **131**(Jul): 1–10.

Nurminen T (1998) Shift work and reproductive health. *Scandinavian Journal of Work, Environment and Health.* **24**(Suppl 3): 28–34.

O'Donnell RD and Eggemeier FT (1986) Workload assessment methodology. In: KR Boff, L Kaufman and JP Thomas (eds) *Handbook of Perception and Human Performance. Vol.11: Cognitive Processes and Performance.* Wiley, New York.

Olsson K, Kandolin I and Kauppinintoropainen K (1990) Stress and coping strategies of 3-shift workers. *Travail Humain.* **53**(2): 175–88.

Reid GB and Nygren TE (1988) The subjective workload assessment technique: a scaling procedure for measuring mental workload. In: P Hancock and N Meshkati (eds) *Human Mental Workload*. Advances in Psychology Series, 52. Elsevier, Amsterdam, pp. 185–218.

Romon-Rousseaux M, Lancry A, Poulet I, Frimat P and Furon D (1987) Effect of protein and carbohydrate snacks on alertness during the night. In: A Oginski, J Pokorski and J Rutenfranz (eds) *Contemporary Advances in Shift Work Research: theoretical and practical aspects in the late eighties*. Krakow Medical Academy. Peter Lang, Frankfurt, pp. 133–41.

Rosa RR *et al.* (1990) Intervention factors for promoting adjustment to nightwork and shiftwork. *Occupational Medicine*. 5(2): 391–415.

Samkoff JS and Jacques CHM (1991) A review of studies concerning the effects of sleep deprivation and fatigue on residents' performance. *Academic Medicine*. 66(11): 687–93.

Scott AJ (1990) *Occupational Medicine: state of the art reviews – shiftwork*. 5(2). Hanley and Belfus, Philadelphia.

Scott AJ and LaDou J (1990) Shiftwork: effects on sleep and health with recommendations for medical surveillance and screening. In: AJ Scott (ed.) *Occupational Medicine: state of the art reviews – shiftwork*. 5(2). Hanley and Belfus, Philadelphia, pp. 273–99.

Smith CS *et al.* (1999) A process model of shiftwork and health. *Journal of Occupational Health Psychology*. 4(3): 207–18.

Smith L *et al.* (1998a) Industrial shift systems in the UK. *Applied Ergonomics*. 29(4): 273–80.

Smith L *et al.* (1998b) Work shift duration: a review comparing eight hour and 12 hour shift systems. *Occupational and Environmental Medicine*. 55(4): 217–29.

Stampi C (1989) Ultrashort sleep/wake patterns and sustained performance. In: DF Dinges and RJ Broughton (eds) *Sleep and Alertness: chronobiological, behavioural and medical aspects of napping*. Raven Press, New York, pp. 139–69.

Suskin N *et al.* (1998) Clinical workload decreases the level of aerobic fitness in housestaff physicians. *Journal of Cardiopulmonary Rehabilitation*. 18(3): 216–20.

Takahashi M, Nakata A, Haratani T, Ogawa Y and Arito H (2003) Post-lunch nap at a worksite to promote daytime alertness in factory workers. *Ergonomics*. 47(9): 1003–13.

Tanz RR and Charrow J (1993) Black clouds. Workload, sleep and resident reputation. *American Journal of Diseases in Children*. 147(5): 579–84.

Tattersall AJ (2000) Workload and task allocation. In: N Chmiel (ed.) *Introduction to Work and Organizational Psychology: a European perspective*. Blackwell, Oxford, ch.8.

Tattersall AJ and Foord PS (1996) An experimental evaluation of instantaneous self-assessment as a measure of workload. *Ergonomics*. 39(5): 740–8.

Taylor E (1994) *The Evaluation of a Counselling Service for Shift Workers*. (Unpublished PhD thesis) MRC ESRC Social and Applied Psychology Unit, University of Sheffield.

Tepas DI and Mahan RP (1989) The many meanings of sleep. *Work and Stress*. 3(1): 93–102.

Thapar A (1989) Psychiatric disorder in the medical profession. *British Journal of Hospital Medicine*. 42(6): 480–3.

Torsvall L *et al.* (1989) Sleep on the night shift: 24 hour EEG monitoring of spontaneous sleep/wake behaviour. *Psychophysiology*. 26(3): 352–8.

Tov N, Rubin AH and Lavie P (1995) Effects of workload on residents' sleep duration: objective documentation. *Israeli Journal of Medical Sciences*. 31(7): 417–22.

Vaillant GE, Sobowale NC and McArthur C (1972) Some psychologic vulnerabilities of physicians. *New England Journal of Medicine*. 287(8): 372–5.

Vassallo DJ *et al.* (1992) Introduction of a partial shift system for house officers in a teaching hospital. *BMJ*. 305(6860): 1005–8.

Veltman JA and Gaillard AW (1996) Physiological indices of workload in a simulated flight task. *Biological Psychology*. 42(3): 323–42.

Volger A *et al.* (1988) Common free time of family members under different shift systems. *Applied Ergonomics.* **19**(3): 213–18.

Waterhouse J, Folkard S and Minors D (1992) *Shift work, Health and Safety: An overview of the scientific literature 1978–1990.* HSE, HMSO, London.

Webb WB and Levy CM (1984) Effects of spaced and repeated total sleep deprivation. *Ergonomics.* **27**(1): 45–58.

Wilkinson RT (1968) Sleep deprivation: performance tests for partial and selective sleep deprivation. *Progress in Clinical Psychology.* **8**: 28–43.

Wilkinson RT, Tyler PD and Varey CA (1975) Duty hours of young hospital doctors: effects on the quality of work. *Journal of Occupational Psychology.* **48**(4): 219–29.

Wilson GF and Eggemeier FT (1991) Psychophysiological assessment of workload in multi-task environments. In: DL Damos (ed.) *Multiple-task Performance.* Taylor and Francis, London, pp. 329–60.

Conclusions

Why did we do this?

Generally speaking, doctors do not perform poorly simply because they lack knowledge or skills or because they are lazy. Why do intelligent individuals who have been sufficiently talented and motivated to qualify as doctors underperform? How can the causes of poor performance be identified, remedied and prevented?

The aim of this work is to understand in more detail why the performance of a small minority of doctors does not meet the expectations of patients, the public, colleagues or employers.

This is a complex set of questions. Not surprisingly, the interpretation of the evidence and its extrapolation to the performance of doctors are also complex.

The factors fall into two broad categories:

1 Individual factors:
   - physical health
   - psychological health
   - personality and attitudes
   - education, training and continuing professional development.
2 Factors associated with work:
   - climate and culture
   - team working
   - leadership
   - workload, sleep and shift work.

The study of each group of factors exposes a general lack of evidence. It also raises a number of important policy and research questions.

Individual factors

Doctors' physical and psychological health may have a significant impact on professional performance. Health problems are underdiagnosed and often poorly managed, not least when doctors choose to self-diagnose and self-treat. Should guidance about the dangers of doctors managing their own and their families' health be publicised or enforced more widely? Should, as suggested in Chapter 1, occupational health assessments include more objective assessment of health, disease and function? Airline pilots are required to have health assessments on a 6-monthly cycle. Just as an unhealthy pilot can put airline passengers at risk, so too can an unhealthy doctor put patients and the public at risk. Should doctors have regular health checks? Should their work hours be more strictly controlled? To what extent does stress at work and at home affect performance? How can stress be reduced?

Being well developed and unlikely to change in adult life, personality is a major factor in professional performance. Characteristics such as the 'Big Five' (Conscientiousness, Emotional Stability, Openness, Extraversion and Agreeableness) are associated with success in professional and business activities. However, extremes of these characteristics, including 'overplayed strengths', can be causes for concern. For example, too much or too little confidence leads to problems in decision making, a task integral to the practice of medicine. Excessively high self-esteem may be associated with aggression.

Many of these traits are apparent early in adulthood. To what extent should they be taken into account in selection of medical students? If we are able to predict a reasonable likelihood of derailment in a young person who wishes to become a doctor, is it fair on either the individual or society (which pays the bulk of the costs of medical education in the UK and which will ultimately bear the results of a poorly performing doctor) to select that person for medical school?

Such a question is complex. The evidence base on the efficacy of selection and prediction using standardised instruments is far from watertight. Furthermore, medicine is a multifaceted profession and requires a range of personality types, talents and interests to fill the many roles. The question of personality assessment in medical student recruitment deserves further debate.

Drugs and alcohol misuse are common but underdiagnosed. Should screening be routine? If so, should it be for all doctors, for those in 'safety-critical' jobs or only for those with alleged performance problems? Again the arguments are complex but, if we know that drugs and alcohol cause impaired performance and that their use is prevalent in the medical profession, isn't there a duty to address the problem?

Perhaps more importantly, what can employers, colleagues and educators do to moderate the causes of drug and alcohol misuse, for example by reducing stress at work, increasing awareness of the problems and providing support and effective medical intervention when problems arise? If, as the evidence seems to suggest, about three-quarters of doctors misusing alcohol can be rehabilitated, would screening be cost-effective?

Impaired cognitive function has a number of possible causes. It is underdiagnosed and may be concealed by the effective social and interpersonal skills typical of educated people. It seems that, to date, there is no specific and sensitive screening test available and that, if it is suspected in an occupational health examination, assessment by a neuropsychologist or neuropsychiatrist is necessary. Further research is necessary to describe the prevalence and causes of cognitive impairment in doctors.

That education, including the teaching and learning of professional values and role-modelling, affects performance is self-evident. However, the early signs of trainees in difficulty ('disappearing act', low work-rate, ward rage, rigidity, bypass syndrome, career problems and insight failure, etc.) are less well known. Many of these characteristics will be familiar. How can we better use available information to identify colleagues in difficulty and to ensure effective, early intervention before patients and the public are put at risk?

Factors associated with work

There is a conflict in the NHS between the 'transactional' culture of leadership by control, performance monitoring and league tables, etc. and the potential benefits of a more 'transformational' approach in which leaders encourage creativity and participation. To what extent do these forces, which sometimes oppose each other, affect performance and what can be done about it?

The chapters on climate and culture, team working, leadership and workload highlight the relationship between the context in which a person works and the outcomes of their work. There are indications that leadership culture affects performance in healthcare. For example, there is evidence to suggest that fewer patients die when they are looked after by well-managed teams, which are also more cost-effective. Similarly, in manufacturing, organisational climate predicts 29% of variation in productivity and profitability. How can these factors be measured and, where necessary, changed?

The effects of workload on performance are increasingly clear and, in the UK at least, there is a move towards recognition of this, with reduction of the workload expectations of doctors in training and reconfiguration of work patterns for senior doctors. However, total hours worked are not the only influence on performance, and new work patterns often impose different demands such as increased shift work and more intensive technical work. There is no clear evidence as to the extent to which managing workload and fatigue is taken seriously in the NHS.

What did we find?

Prevention

The old adage 'prevention is better than cure' is just as important in the management of a doctor's performance as it is elsewhere in healthcare.

The evidence on prevention is weak. This is not surprising, since prevention is only possible once there is clarity about the factors that influence (poor) performance which need to be modified. The development of robust prevention strategies would require an evidence base followed by research on interventions to determine what strategies prevented what, how and for whom. This should become part of the research agenda.

For the moment, discussion on prevention must centre, as much of this book does, on an extrapolation of our understanding of the factors that might influence performance. The discussion centres on three levels – organisations, systems and the individual.

Chapter 7 demonstrates how organisational culture and climate influence the effectiveness and wellbeing of a workforce, with some evidence that certain cultures influence the outcomes and safety of healthcare for patients. A positive organisational culture can therefore be seen as playing a part in the prevention of poor performance. It can be argued that there are fewer performance problems in organisations where the workforce is valued and where there is effective leadership. It is likely that, when individual performance problems begin to emerge in a constructive and supportive work climate, early, effective action is taken to address the problems and mitigate their effects.

Prevention of poor performance is one of a range of responsibilities of every senior manager and policy maker including, in particular, the evidence suggests, chief executives and Board members.

At a systems level, the development and support of effective teams have an effect on performance. Properly constituted teams may therefore be an important preventative factor. There is a substantial literature that points in this direction. The problem seems to be in their implementation in the healthcare workplace. Many healthcare professionals think that they work in teams when the evidence suggests they actually work in groups with only a partial, often implicit, agreement about common goals. Moreover, in the National Health Service (NHS), work is rarely constructed around teams who stay together for particular tasks for much of their time. Even if people do work in a group, they are usually also members of other small groups which may have different goals.

There are some pragmatic steps that can be taken to improve the performance of individuals in healthcare teams. Training in teamwork, in what teams are and in what they are not should improve both team leadership and individual team member performance. Evidence cited in this book suggests that improving inter-group co-operation through understanding each other's roles, shared objectives and participation in decision making may also be effective in improving performance. Such training could be an important element in preventing poor group and individual performance.

At the individual level, successful prevention appears to be mainly related to educational and human resources interventions. There is surprisingly little available information on the impact on professional performance of medical student selection procedures. If extremes of personality type are associated with subsequent professional difficulties, should personality testing be part of medical school selection?

There is a suggestion that transfer of information from universities to subsequent educational supervisors might be a useful tool in the early identification of problems, perhaps offering the chance to prevent or remediate in time to mitigate performance problems. Transition from student to doctor has been shown to be a difficult period in professional development. Support systems for individuals, for example through improved education, supervision and assessment now being introduced into the early years of practice in the United Kingdom, should promote good professional practice and limit the likelihood of performance problems.

Lastly, the new appraisal systems in the NHS, together with General Medical Council proposals for revalidation, may also identify opportunities for secondary, if not primary, prevention of performance problems.

Identification

Underperformance can be caused by incompetence, but other causes are equally likely. When problems arise, it is important to take a wide view and to consider the whole range of causes of underperformance discussed in these chapters.

How should one approach the problem of a doctor who appears to be under-performing? On the basis of the evidence presented in this book, we propose the following framework.

First of all, is the doctor physically or psychologically ill? Is there any indication that alcohol or substance misuse might be a factor? Is there any evidence that the doctor is cognitively impaired, for example by Alzheimer's disease or brain injury? Excellent occupational health services are not universal, but a good occupational health or psychiatric assessment should be considered at an early stage. Suspected cognitive impairment may require expert assessment by a neuropsychologist or neuropsychiatrist.

Is the doctor's behaviour self-defeating or counterproductive? Assessment by an occupational or clinical psychologist may help to identify the problem(s) and indicate whether an intervention such as cognitive behaviour therapy or psychotherapy is likely to be effective. Does the doctor's personality and behaviour make him or her better suited for alternative employment?

Medical practice is characterised by stress and people respond to stress in different ways. Is stress affecting performance? Could racism, sexism or other discrimination be a factor? Enquiries must be carried out with sensitivity by the most appropriate person in the circumstances. Good managers and Human Resources departments can identify and understand the pressures on members of their workforce and manage them accordingly.

Are problems related to deficiencies in training? Has the doctor missed out on critical parts of professional development or been exposed to counterproductive role models? The educational needs of a poorly performing doctor should always be considered, bearing in mind that education is not a panacea and that goals should be explicit and realistic.

To what extent does the presenting problem of a poorly performing doctor reflect wider problems within a team, department or organisation? An individual may be a scapegoat for a dysfunctional team. The climate and culture of an organisation are major factors affecting the performance of its staff. Factors such as reorganisation, bullying, poor teamwork and lack of leadership are not uncommon. Although such causes of underperformance should be apparent to those responsible for managing staff, they may not be. Indeed, even if those responsible possess the necessary skills and experience, the people responsible for sorting out problems may be part of the problem or too closely involved to be objective.

In clinical practice, diagnosis should precede treatment. The management of poor performance is the same. Causes should be identified first.

Remediation

To remediate can be defined as 'to correct, redress or rectify something that is at fault or error'. It may therefore be an unhelpful or inappropriate term when used in relation to factors that are not necessarily due to any fault or error on the part of the individual. It may be more constructive to broaden the term to include not only correction but also alleviation. For example, although correction of cognitive impairment may not be possible, its impact may be alleviated.

Evidence about effective remediation is limited. In some areas there may be several proven routes to successful remediation; in other areas the evidence is either conflicting or missing.

The development of remedial work needs to focus on improved co-operation between experts in the problem, for example between neuropsychologists and occupational medicine specialists and employers. Currently some of these links are weak. Stronger professional relationships between a range of disciplines may help to ensure that the doctor is referred to the right source of specialist help.

Organisational interventions, for example changing ways of organising practice and training, building team relationships, etc., seem to be effective in reducing staff stress levels and litigation. It may also be important to provide other interventions, including good assessment, counselling, psychotherapy and occupational health.

With regard to psychological factors, the quality of evidence on the ability to change behaviour is generally poor. Behaviours and cognitions are thought to be easier to change than personality. The ability to change requires self-esteem, insight, motivation and support. Teaching about personality types and their implication within teams may help doctors to recognise the impact of their behaviour. There is mixed evidence about the potential for changing specific behaviours: Type A behaviour and narcissism, for example, are not easy to change, but perfectionism may be altered by teaching good coping skills. Self-criticism (an important factor in the ability to respond to feedback) can possibly be altered by psychodynamic intervention. Much of this remains at the level of opinion and experience rather than being supported by robust research evidence.

There is an urgent need for more systematic research into the effects of different interventions on the ability to change behaviour. How much do we really understand about why people change their behaviour? What can we learn from other relevant fields of work such as addiction treatment, and theories of motivation and change? Answers to these questions could help to ensure that remediation and intervention efforts are directed in an appropriate and cost-effective way.

When it comes to factors associated with work, the findings about remediability are mixed. Most clear-cut are the effects of workload on performance. In the UK at least, there is some move towards recognition of this, with reduction of workload expectations of doctors in training. We don't know what the effects of reconfiguration of work patterns for senior doctors will be. However, the total number of hours worked is not the only influence on performance. New work patterns often require different demands such as increased shift work and more intensive technical work. The effects of workload, sleep loss and shift patterns should be alleviated by a number of factors including changing working hours, training, counselling, increasing awareness of personal coping strategies and changing aspects of the working environment. Evidence of effectiveness is conflicting, however; there is no evidence that any one intervention has a significant effect. To what extent is it possible to harness individual natural strengths when planning work and designing rotas? To what extent would it be acceptable to colleagues if, for example, a doctor were to be excused night work because of extreme 'morningness' (*see* Chapter 10)? Training to cope with shift work and complex, high intensity work is possible and can be seen as both a preventative and remedial strategy in performance. There is, however, no clear evidence as to the extent to which managing workload and fatigue is taken seriously in the NHS.

In the area of education and training, remediability is more clear-cut than in other areas. Evidence is largely centred on helping poor performers to develop a deeper learning style, better coping strategies for stress, and insight into personal deficiencies through training. It is generally accepted that poor insight is difficult to remedy.

To be effective, remediation should be supported by an educational framework that supports education and training through increased supervision and regular feedback. We need to understand more about the longer-term success and sustainability of educational interventions. How can we ensure that organisations are investing wisely when supporting remedial programmes? How does an organisation decide when and whether to continue investing in such support for a doctor? Findings on psychological factors and learning styles clearly indicate that remedial programmes for doctors must be appropriately tailored to their personality type, disposition, and learning style. Attending courses, for example, will not suit doctors who learn better through more 'hands-on', practical activity. Implications of cultural differences in learning styles need to be better understood, as do the effects of the aging process on ability to learn in later life. The emphasis on reflective learning in UK medical training and education may be challenging for doctors trained in a more didactic culture.

The work on organisational culture and climate, team working and leadership highlights important common themes in relation to remediation. Enhanced team working boosts organisational performance – but effects on the performance of individual doctors still need to be better understood. It is difficult to determine from the research whether effects on performance can be remedied until we have better qualitative studies of how they actually impact on an individual doctor's performance. Future work is necessary, including on successful strategies to remediate dysfunctional teams.

Leadership is central to effective team working as well as to the culture and climate or the organisation. The personality of the leader will have an inevitable impact at every level – individual, team and organisation. Research evidence on psychological factors suggests that doctors who assume (or are elected into) leadership roles are more likely to struggle because of interpersonal difficulties, failure to adapt to change or complexity, or failure to build and motivate a team than from their lack of technical expertise or knowledge. This has implications for the selection and training of doctors in leadership positions. It also highlights the importance of providing feedback before the behaviours that cause difficulties become too entrenched.

Ethnicity, diversity and the performance of doctors

There is a substantial and broad-ranging international literature on the impact of ethnicity and diversity on human performance and, to a lesser extent, on the performance of healthcare staff. Much of the literature concludes that inequalities that impact on minority groups exist around the world, in the whole field of human endeavour.

In the United Kingdom, a number of commentaries suggest that inequalities, sometimes linked to abuse, have a significant impact on the work of healthcare professionals, including doctors, and that this can lead to underperformance. Clearly this is an important area that needs further research to provide evidence on which improvements could be based.

The range of evidence, from research studies to public policy commentary, leads us to suggest that when considering issues relating to professional performance it is important to consider carefully and take account of the possibility of unequal treatment of any individual or group.

Scope

The study of poor professional performance in healthcare is in its infancy. Although this book is about doctors, it is probable that many of the factors apply to other health professionals, including dentists, nurses and others. The book also refers particularly to practice in the UK. Poorly performing or impaired physicians are not uniquely a UK problem and there is much important and successful work going on around the world including in Canada, the USA, New Zealand, Australia, Ireland

and South Africa. We hope that this book is a useful contribution to the world literature and that it will complement work published in other countries.

More immediately, we hope that the book will inform those responsible for the management of doctors' performance and career guidance as well as those responsible for planning and managing health services.

Index